HEALING GRAVES'

ROADMAP TO GETTING YOUR LIFE AND VITALITY BACK

This book contains advice and information related to health care. It should supplement rather than replace the advice of your doctor or another trained health professional. If you suspect or know that you have a health problem, it is recommended that you seek your physician's advice before embarking on any health or medical program or treatment. All efforts have been made to ensure the accuracy of the information of this book as of publication. The publisher and the author disclaim liability for any medical outcomes that may occur because of applying the methods suggested in this book.

www.healinggravesbook.com

Author photo: Camilla Lindqvist
Design: Katapult
ISBN 9789151969930

CONTENT

To my readers,
may you be successful in taking back the
power over your own health.

WELCOME TO HEALING GRAVES'

One morning in October 2014, I woke up and everything felt grey inside of me. Life did not feel worth living anymore. At first, I thought it was a reaction to events earlier in the year. In January, my mother had died after a long time of being ill, and a month later I had my second child. It was, to say the least, a roller coaster ride of negative and positive life events. In the autumn, I therefore thought the grief after my mother had caught up with me. After a while I felt better, but a voice inside me still said that something was wrong. I booked an appointment with the health center to check the symptoms. I was lucky, the doctor immediately ordered blood samples, including for thyroid function. I have understood afterwards when talking to others, that it is not certain you are thoroughly investigated if you come in with the symptoms I had, more concerning mental health. A few weeks after the blood test, I was diagnosed with Graves' disease. At diagnosis, there is about a 40 percent chance of eventually being declared cured from Graves'. To increase my chances of getting well, I made lifestyle changes to help self-healing. Diet and gut health were tools for self-healing. Using an elimination diet, I created a personal healing diet. My husband and I moved from an energy and money consuming house to free up time for what we value higher: family and friends.

I cleaned out toxins at home, tried various supplements, switched to less stressful work and took several other measures.

It is difficult to point out exactly what did it, maybe all parts have made their contribution, but in the autumn 2016 I stopped all drugs and was declared cured in spring of 2017. Did I feel well? No. Fatigue was my biggest problem. With my own hormones back, I had hoped that some of my symptoms would go away. I got a transient feeling of being stronger physically, but it soon subsided. My disappointment was enormous, who would help me now - my blood tests were perfect, but in terms of well-being I had reached the bottom. Today, I finally feel restored, thanks to further lifestyle changes which you will learn about in this book. It was a long way to go, but today I enjoy life to the fullest again. Since I have a background as a Master of Biomedicine from Karolinska Institute. and am a science and health journalist - it came naturally to write a book on improving Graves' with lifestyle. As I began the research for the book, imagine my surprise when I realised that there is so much information patients never get at the time of diagnosis. My instinct as a journalist was also to interview the sharpest health experts to draw from their knowledge and wisdom. The interviews are included in the book, and I know you will benefit from their clinical pearls as much as I did. I hope that it will now be useful for you through this book.

May you be successful in taking your health into your own hands!

What we wish someone had told us at the time of diagnosis

We often feel very lonely and lost when we receive our diagnosis. If you keep an eye out, there are many wise women who have had the disease that we may ask advice from. Here, some of them share what they wish they had known at diagnosis.

Veronica: "I wish someone had told me what it really means to have surgery to remove a thyroid gland and not just say," It is easy all you have to do is take your medication and you will feel good". Personally, I had many problems as my body does not do well on synthetic T4. I had to find a doctor who understands and listens to the patient. That is difficult."

Emma: "I wish I had known Graves' is not black or white. Be sure to think for yourself and listen not only to what the doctors say. Also, you may get different advice depending on your doctor. Search for facts yourself and do not give up. Everything will be OK. You do not have to remove your thyroid gland, you can get well anyway. Medicine alone does not have to be the only way, adding diet and lifestyle changes can be the right thing for you."

Hanna: "I think doctors downplay the disease. I became so ill that I was about to die, and was lucky that the first doctor was good, but when she quit it got much worse. After 4 months, I switched to a private doctor who listens to me. It has now been 2 years and 7 months since the time of diagnosis and I am still far from well. The first doctor said that patience is the most important thing to equip yourself with in abundance, including for those closest to you. Then she invited the people close to me for an introduction and offered to talk to the employer. This was great and I wish everyone would get this support. After that, the occupational health service had a review with my then boss, and scared the life out of him. It has made it easier for me on all fronts. I think otherwise it would have been difficult for my family when my life was put on hold. Also, accept for yourself that everyone else's life goes on."

Magdalena: "Number one: information, and not only what your doctor tells you, it was thanks to Facebook groups and Dr Google I could gather knowledge about the disease and push for all blood markers to be tested and not just standard the standard ones, be persistent. Number Two: I recommend that you change your diet even though most endocrinologists say there is not enough evidence for that - but it makes a difference in your body. Try to eat as clean food as possible, the Autoimmune Protocol or go for 80/20, do the best you can, it makes a difference. Begin exercising – it makes a big difference. Use a pedometer or heart rate monitor and start walking and slowly build up depending on your heart rate and stamina, do yoga."

Lisa: "I was really ill when I was diagnosed. It has been 3 years and I have not recovered yet. When I got the disease, I would have wanted to know more information about all the symptoms and that recovery can take a long time. I wish that both I and my family had received information that the disease not only affects the thyroid gland, heart and possibly the eyes. In addition, I would have liked to hear that it can be a long-term course with effects on muscles, brain, insomnia and energy levels. We got the impression that after one to three weeks of medical treatment, the symptoms would be reduced. The hospital's endocrinology department has been an excellent support during the process. For the past year and a half, I have received invaluable help with rehabilitation through a physiotherapist."

Annica: "I was diagnosed with Graves' just over 10 years ago, in December 2009. This was followed by medication for 18 months. But the disease came back, and I had surgery on my thyroid in 2013. After that, it has been a long journey to feel better, but in recent years I have felt better again even though I still have some symptoms left that come and go.

At the time of diagnosis, I wish that someone would have said that this can be lifelong, it can become chronic and is something that you may have to live with. I remember a doctor who said: "you will be completely healthy", and I believed in it, but that was not true.

Lifestyle changes are individual, but for me it is a lot about diet. I have many problems with my gut and have been diagnosed with chronic gastritis. Another thing I think affects symptoms is stress, so you really need to minimize it in your life. Exercise is an important part, but not too hard exercise. For example, I cannot run because then I feel terrible afterwards, but yoga, walking and strength training work very well."

PART ONE - ABOUT THE DISEASE

What did you learn about Graves' at the time of diagnosis? Some of us remember nothing from the first visits to the doctor or what was said there. We were far too affected by the disease. Alternatively, as the women in the previous section describe, information that Graves' can have a deep and lasting impact on our lives is sometimes left out. If you have noticed that you do not feel as vital as before, you are not alone. But there are many things you can do to activate your body's self-healing mechanisms.

CHAPTER 1
WHERE DID QUALITY OF LIFE GO?

When we suffer from Graves' disease, we have a lower quality of life and this may continue as the years go by. 25 percent of us with Graves' still eight years after diagnosis experience that we have not fully recovered. The list of symptoms can be long and many concern our mental well-being. It is not a given that you heal spontaneously from Graves', as both patients and doctors often believe. A common way to look at Graves' is: "Fix the hormone levels, then the symptoms dissolve". But studies show that even if your hormone levels have been normal for a long time, the disease can linger on in the shape of symptoms and reduced quality of life. A research group writes in one article: "Doctors often assume that Graves' is transient and that when a patient reaches normal thyroid hormone levels, the same health and quality of life is restored as before the disease. On the contrary, our results show that Graves' can be a chronic disease with effects on the patient's well-being, both in the short and long term…"

Women with Graves' are offered more or less the same treatment options, although we are all unique. The way forward is to embrace that uniqueness and create a plan that is tailored to you. The approach in this book is based on lifestyle changes. That does not mean that the medical treatment is not an important foundation in feeling better, but when we continue to have stubborn symptoms after Graves' - using lifestyle as a way of feeling better is a goldmine.

In this book, we look at some aspects of health that are affected by the disease, each of which lower the quality of life. You will also create a personal roadmap to healing with the power to improve the quality of life. Your roadmap will help you:

- Reduce inflammation
- Calm the immune system
- Balance brain and nervous system
- Restore nutritional balance
- Get more energy
- Build muscle and bones
- Acceptance as a way of transforming your view of your health.

You will learn how you can notice which parts of the body are hardest hit by the disease. Then you will create your own roadmap of your healing. Direct your efforts during recovery there. Our genetics and lifestyle look different, your map will be unique - just like you are.

Can Graves' be cured?

The answer is a resounding: Yes! Research shows that eight years after diagnosis, it is possible for about 40 percent of you to have a thyroid that is producing hormones and take no hormonal replacement or antithyroid medication. Graves' can have one episode and then calm down to disappear for the rest of your life. The body is fantastic at healing itself. If you above that, create a personal healing roadmap, you have every possibility for a healing rate of more than 40 percent. Here you will learn what research says about who gets well and what you can do to improve your chances. Keep in mind that for those of us who are not cured, the reversal of the symptoms is fully possible. You can regain your vitality and quality of life, have more energy, feel less stressed and just plain be happier about your life. And even though you are not cured, you can lower the markers of active disease to give your body the possibility to regenerate and have vibrant health.

What is health?

> “Health is a state of complete physical, mental and social well-being, not just the absence of disease and disability."
>
> World Health Organization (WHO)

A blood test cannot tell you, or anyone else, if you are feeling good or bad. Many of us with Graves' have experienced this. You know best how you feel. It is possible to have "perfect" hormone values and still feel in poor condition. And conversely, it is possible to have a blood test that shows "bad" values, even if you have an experience of feeling good.

Doctors and patients often believe, as we have seen before, that Graves' is a transient disease, that when the thyroid hormones show normal values again, the quality of life is also restored. Unfortunately, this is not the case, but well-being may continue to be affected for many years to come. There is a difference between being cured and being recovered. This means that the diagnostic criteria for the disease may no longer fit you, T4 is normal and so is TSH, with no treatment for the thyroid gland. But you are still dragged down by the suites after the disease. In short, you still feel like you have not gotten your life and vitality back.

The reasons the patients themselves usually state that they do not feel recovered are: fatigue, eye-related problems, problems with the hormone replacement treatment (usually T4 in synthetic form) or other treatment related to the disease and worries about living with a chronic disease which may recur.

Measuring quality of life is better than taking blood samples to find out how affected you are by your disease. Measuring patients' quality of life is used in healthcare, and many believe that an excellent quality of life is the only reasonable goal for a treatment. It is about how you experience your quality of life.

If you have Graves' ophthalmopathy, the eye disease associated with Graves', you are likely to experience a lower quality of life than others with Graves'. In measurements of quality of life. patients in this group mainly get lower scores on questions about how they feel about their physical health and their appearance, than others with Graves'.

Although we humans function similarly purely biochemically, there are often significant differences. Today, the treatment we are offered use a one size fits all approach. If thyroid replacement therapy does not help you have the quality of life you desire, then what can you do? We should then remind ourselves that we all have access to a great opportunity. It can be individually adapted and varied endlessly: lifestyle. You and your friend may both have had Graves' but probably need different roadmaps for sleep, food, recovery, and movement to achieve the experience of health and a high quality of life.

You are the expert of you

A good medical treatment is the basis for recovery and cannot be underestimated. When the thyroid hormones are normalized, the body can often rebalance itself and we are restored. In addition, there are indications that the drug treatment itself helps to calm the immune system. But we have seen that far from everyone is restored. If this applies to you, here is your chance of becoming the expert of your own health. Because – and let us be honest, no one is going to care as deeply about your healing as you do. In addition, no one knows your body as well as you do.

The importance of tailoring a healthy lifestyle for experiencing an excellent quality of life is not news to you. When we eat, exercise and sleep well, we feel better. But using the lifestyle to recover when we suffer from reduced quality of life because of illness may be unfamiliar.

For other diseases known to lower our quality of life, such as cancer and Parkinson's disease, lifestyle factors have proven to be important. Cancer patients with a healthier lifestyle also have a higher quality of life than those with the same serious illness who live less healthily. One study examined the effects of anti-inflammatory diets in Parkinson's disease and found that those who followed the diet had fewer symptoms of their disease and increased quality of life. This is so encouraging to us all.

Graves' can be an opportunity to find out what a healing lifestyle looks like for you. To get to know your body and mind in ways you did not before. It is time to be curious and ask yourself the question:

How may I, in my current situation, use my lifestyle to improve my quality of life?

CHAPTER 2

WHAT IS GRAVES' DISEASE?

You probably know that the thyroid gland controls your metabolism. More thyroid hormone means faster metabolism and less means slower. Therefore, hyperthyroidism often leads to weight loss and hypothyroidism to weight gain. The thyroid gland affects many aspects of our health and is also important for the heart, muscles and bones, gastrointestinal function, fertility and brain health.

The gland is butterfly-shaped and located at the front of the neck. The production of hormones in the thyroid gland is controlled from the brain, or more specifically a part of the brain called the hypothalamus. It keeps track of our internal environment and sends orders to another part of the brain, the pituitary gland, if something needs to be balanced. The hypothalamus can perceive the levels of thyroid hormone in the blood, and if you need more, it sends a request to the pituitary gland in the form of thyrotropin-releasing hormone (TRH).

The brain can also perceive an increased need for thyroid hormone in the form of stressors, physiological or emotional, and then increase the release of TRH. A physiological stressor can be cold, then the body wants to increase metabolism to generate heat.

An emotional stressor can be the loss of a loved one. In the long run, however, stress is inhibitory to the thyroid glands' release of hormones. On the signal of TRH, the pituitary produces thyroid-stimulating hormone (TSH), which binds to receptors for TSH in the thyroid. The thyroid cells then form T4 (thyroxine) from the amino acid tyrosine and the mineral iodine. However, T4 is inactive and must be converted to T3, with the ability to activate its receptors in the cells. 20 percent of T4 is converted to T3 in the thyroid. The rest is sent out into the blood stream and is converted in the liver. To some extent, T3 can also be formed in the intestines and brain. Receptors for thyroid hormone are found in the heart, kidneys, fat cells, muscles and brain. Many receptors for T3 are found in the brain. No wonder Graves' often has consequences for how we feel mentally.

Normally, the levels of T4 and T3 are carefully regulated in the blood. When they increase, a signal is sent to the brain to decrease TSH, which results in the thyroid gland producing less hormone.

Glossary thyroid gland

TRH - Thyrotropin-releasing hormone. Excreted from the brain and causes the pituitary gland to produce TSH. TRH can also affect the nervous system and the brain.

TSH - Thyroid-stimulating hormone causes the thyroid gland to produce T4.

T4 - Thyrxine, inactive thyroid hormone. Converted mainly in the liver to the active form T3.

T3 – Triiodothyronine, active thyroid hormone, which together with other hormones balances our internal environment, including our metabolism.

rT3 - Stands for reverse T3 and is an inactive form of the hormone. This can increase when the body wants to protect us from stress.

Adrenaline and noradrenaline - Stress hormones with rapid effects in the body. Gets you ready for flight or flight. T3 enhances the effects of adrenaline in the body.

Cortisol - Vital stress hormone that monitors blood sugar and the immune system. Under normal conditions, cortisol and T3 are in a fine-tuned balance with each other.

TRAb - Thyroid-stimulating hormone receptor antibodies. Elevated in Graves' disease, which provides constant stimulation of the thyroid gland. They can cause damage to the thyroid gland and therefore contribute to hypothyroidism.

TPOAb - These antibodies attack Thyroid peroxidase and interfere with the formation of T4 hormone, contributing to damage of the tissue and may contribute to lower function of the thyroid.

Common in Hashimoto's hypothyroidism which is the most common autoimmune thyroid disease, but many with Graves' also have high levels of these antibodies.

TGAb - These antibodies attack thyroglobulin, which is a protein in the thyroid gland. Common mainly in Hashimoto's hypothyroidism but also in many with Graves'.

Receptor - The cell's receiver for a messenger, often a hormone. Stimulation of a receptor then has an effect in the cell.

Interview with Ove Törring, Associate Professor, former Senior Lecturer and Chief Physician: The recovery may take time

Ove Törring, Associate Professor, former Senior Lecturer and Chief Physician, has treated thousands of patients with Graves' and researched the disease since the 1980s. His studies have become influential on for example guidelines for treatment of Graves' in many countries, including the United States. Ove Törring's current research covers the long-term consequences of Graves' and the latest studies concern the long-term quality of life in patients with Graves'. These studies have gained much interest, perhaps especially because they have shown that those who have received radioiodine have a poorer quality of life than patients with other treatments.

Ove Törring says that patients with Graves' disease have a poorer quality of life compared to others. He and his research colleagues have seen this up to 17 years after diagnosis.

"We do not know exactly why that is, but possibly something important changes in the brain with the disease. Something that is difficult to restore. Even if patients with Graves' disease feel better after treatment and over time, we know that the hyperthyroidism can recur if the thyroid remains and the impact of the disease can be lifelong. It can also take time to recover, having patience for at least one year after diagnosis before feeling better is often necessary."

Patients with radioiodine treatment also have a higher risk of poorer quality of life.

"We do not know exactly why, I wish we had more research on it. What we know is that patients who receive radioiodine are often older and therefore may have other diseases as well which may have played a role when radioiodine treatment was chosen for them. One could speculate that their comorbidity may explain the lower quality of life in the long term but we have adjusted the data for confounders such as age and comorbidity but the result were the same. Radioiodine also temporarily raises TRAb and can aggravate or cause Graves' ophthalmopathy, which in itself is associated with lower quality of life."

Some patients with Graves' can recognise themselves in descriptions of what it is like to have burnout. Ove says:

"Graves' is not the same as burnout, many symptoms are different. But there are overlaps, including increased stress sensitivity that can last a lifetime. Severe longstanding stress can cause Graves' which I have seen many times. A stressful work situation or other psychological stress can lead to the onset of the disease."

How to fine-tune the treatment

"The treatment of Graves′ disease most often imply that the thyroid hormone production is absent (hypothyroidism) after radioiodine, as in the US, or by surgical treatment. Even after medical treatment, primarily preferred in Europe, 40 percent of our patients in the end needed lifelong replacement therapy with thyroid hormone. Most often adjusting of the replacement dose after treatment may be necessary. However, there can be benefits to changing the dose in smaller steps than usual.

In the beginning, you need to go fast with increases of Levothyroxine until you find the right dose. Then keep in mind that the dose may need adjusting in the future. The dose that was right after 6 months may not be right at all after one year. When the optimal thyroxine dose needs to be found and calibrated, it is best to change the dose in small steps. It can be about 25 or 50 mcg Levothyroxine per week, and then you wait for two months and see how the symptoms change before making an assessment if a new adjustment is needed.

Danish studies have shown that we are all born with an individual setpoint between T4 and TSH. When you begin a hormone replacement therapy, we very seldom know your body's setpoint, i.e. the balance between T4 and TSH, before you became ill. Therefore, it is important to be open to adjusting the treatment and be prepared that small changes over a considerable time may be needed in order to find and mimic this setpoint."

To know when it is time to fine tune, you can pay attention to your symptoms.

"Symptoms of too much hormone replacement are like those of Graves' disease, but in a lighter version.

- Palpitations
- Irritated
- "The thermostat is set high", you sweat easily
- Bigger appetite for food
- Feel distanced from others. The people around you may notice that you are listening politely, but it is difficult to reach you. And often you do as you please anyway.

I usually ask my patients: If you are out walking and get to a hill you usually have no problems to cope with, do you now feel a larger need of air, become more warm and sweaty from walking up that hill than you used to? That can be a sign of too high dose of hormone of your replacement therapy.

If you have too little hormone substitution, you may experience symptoms similar to those of hypothyroidism, such as:

- Difficulties in finding motivation
- Cold
- Loss of hair
- Lower sex drive
- Difficulties in getting pregnant"

Despite that the recommendations are to use L-thyroxine, natural dessicated Thyroid (NDT) is sometime discussed in the treatment of hypothyroidism. Some patients benefit from it, but it is still unclear how it is best used and difficult for the doctor to monitor.

"I have had a few patients who have had significant benefits from NDT, or dried porcine thyroid gland, but the research does not show that there would be any difference in treatment results with NDT compared to levothyroxine except for slightly lower body weight of the patient. Although most of T4 converts to T3 in the body, a healthy thyroid gland produces a certain amount of T3. Levothyroxine contains only T4, and sometimes the conversion from T3 to T4 is affected. It may very well be so that some patients without any remnant thyroid perhaps have slightly lower T3 than they used to have. Some of these perhaps need the addition of a small dose of T3."

Autoimmune diseases rarely heal, instead they become lifelong. But some of us with Graves' only have one episode and are declared cured.

"The autoimmunity in Graves' is usually lifelong and is known to relapse. Those who have had the disease carry immune cells that can make antibodies against the thyroid gland. These can be aroused, for example, after stress when cortisol increases and the immune system becomes unbalanced. Treatment with block and replace helps the immune system to get a break and the cells can become dormant again, but they are always there. To calm your immune system, be sure to take your medication as directed. If you take it irregularly, the hormones can rise from time to time, which delays the healing process. To permanently get rid of the risk that Graves′ disease will recur the thyroid must be permanently inactivated as it is achieved by radioiodine or surgery (total thyroidectomy). No thyroid-no recurrence."

Resting is necessary for healing

When we are most sick, we may not realize that resting is necessary to heal. We may feel that we do not have time for that. According to Ove Törring, however, rest is crucial to ease your symptoms and help the body to heal.

"The most important thing is to reduce your stress levels. Take your stress sensitivity seriously and try to solve difficult situations you are in. Learn to get better at keeping a healthy distance to things. Many would need to take it easy and appreciate life more. I usually tell my patients, even those with small children, that they should take at least 1 hour for themselves every day where they do not worry about work, making dinner or anything else. Do not make major, important life decisions in the first months after diagnosis.

Optimize your sleep. In Graves' disease the sleep becomes fragmented and you often wake up. This leads to the brain not being allowed to rest sufficiently.

I advise against using various stimulants shortly after the diagnosis was made. In some, alcohol can cause palpitations. Coffee and nicotine agitate the nervous system. If you smoke, you really should quit. It is bad for your health in general, but it also contributes to the increased risk of long-term eye problems related to Graves'. Smoke contains substances that interfere with the function of the thyroid gland as well as nicotine have negative actions on the immune system.

Review your work situation. Unfortunately, patients with Graves' do not get a bandage that shows they are ill. Therefore, provide information to your employer and ask for an easier workload."

*

This is Graves' disease

Every year, 1 in 200 people get Graves' disease. It is also the most common type of hyperthyroidism. To make the diagnosis, elevated levels of T4 or T3 should be present in the blood and 95 percent of the patients have high levels of TRAb (Thyroid-stimulating hormone receptor antibodies).

Some of the most common symptoms of Graves' are:

- Palpitation
- Atrial fibrillations

- Irritability, stress intolerance
- Weight loss
- Diarrhea
- Poor physical and mental strength
- Heat intolerance, sweating
- Restlessness
- Trembling hands

Graves' disease is an autoimmune disease. Autoimmunity occurs when the immune system attacks the body's own tissues. In Graves' disease, the thyroid gland is under attack by antibodies against the TSH receptors. Once TRAb has been formed, they can be converted into three different subtypes. One type, the most well-known, stimulates the thyroid gland to produce hormone in excess, even though too much is already in the blood. There is also one type that causes more cells in the thyroid gland to go through cell death, and the last one blocks the effect of the other two. Blocking TRAb is not so common but can cause hypothyroidism, and when the antibodies are alternately stimulating or blocking, hormone levels fluctuate.

It is also common for the immune system to attack the formation of T4 via elevated antibodies against the enzyme thyroid peroxidase and thyroglobulin.

Thyroglobulin is found in the thyroid gland and binds T4 until there is a signal that more hormone is needed in the blood. Thyroglobulin can also transport and bind the thyroid hormones in the blood, which regulates the amount of free hormone. On your test result from the laboratory, you may have noticed that it says fT4 and fT3. It stands for free T4 and free T3. These are the most interesting thyroid hormone values because only free hormones can influence the cells. The rest of the T4 and T3 in the blood are bound to thyroglobulin but can be released when needed.

When the thyroid hormones increase to harmful levels, the body tries to do what it can to reduce production. The brain often lowers the level of TSH to immeasurable levels in Graves' but it does not matter. The TSH receptors continue to be stimulated by the antibodies. The result is a constant acute stress because the fine-tuning function in the stress response is out of play. When the thyroid hormones are in excess, the body becomes more sensitive to noradrenaline and the adrenal gland releases more cortisol. Your body then behaves as if it is exposed to great threats. These are important reasons we feel bad when we have high levels of thyroid hormones, both physically and mentally.

Up to 50 percent also have Graves' ophthalmopathy. The ophthalmopathy may already be there at the time of diagnosis or occur several years later, even when your thyroid levels are normal. There are TSH receptors in the eye tissue and in Graves' ophthalmopathy, cells from the immune system will migrate into the eye socket. There they start a pro-inflammatory process which leads to increased levels of cytokines (the name of a group of immune messengers), growth factors and inflammation. This activates fat cells and cells that produce supporting tissue, which then form glycosaminoglycans. These can attract water so the eye swells and the outflow of blood from the eye is less effective. More fat cells and cells that produce supporting tissue are formed, resulting in greater volume of eye tissue. Patients with ophthalmopathy have one or more of the following symptoms:

- Feeling of grit and irritation in the eyes

- Feeling of pressure behind the eyes
- Increased tear flow
- Varying visual acuity
- Stiffness during eye movements
- Double vision.

Some women also experience symptoms from skin. This is called Graves' dermopathy, and they may suffer the following symptoms:

- Red, swollen skin, usually on the shins and tops of the feet.
- Skin texture may be like that of an orange peel.

Doctors may also refer to the condition as pretibial myxedema.

Treatment options in Graves'

While this is not a book mainly on the medical treatment of Graves', but a book about how to heal using your lifestyle, a few words on treatment options are necessary.

In many countries, antithyroid drugs that block the thyroid from making excess hormone are first line of treatment.

- Methimazole, available in US, Asia and Europe. Has antioxidant properties.
- Carbimazole, available mostly in Europe. Is an inactive form of methimazole.
- Propylthiouracil (PTU), available in US, Asia and Europe. The metabolic effect lasts for 12 to 24 hours, and this means that PTU be taken 2 to 3 times per day.

Either the production is partially blocked, or an approach called "block and replace" is used. The partial block allows your thyroid gland to cover your hormonal needs, while the "block and replace" completely shuts down production. "Block and replace" requires the addition of thyroid hormones in the form of hormonal replacement therapy. The treatment usually lasts for about 12-18 months before discontinuing the antithyroid drugs to see how the thyroid gland manages on its own. For about half of all women, the autoimmune process has then calmed down, and the thyroid can produce enough hormones to meet your needs, without slipping into hyperthyroidism. Perhaps the standard time period for using antithyroid drugs will be extended, since studies show that more women may go into remission if the antithyroid drugs are sustained for a longer period. In addition, women with Graves' ophthalmopathy, the eye disease common in Graves', and a severe hyperthyroidism difficult to treat might benefit from maintaining a dose low of antithyroid drugs for an extended time period. One study concluded that these women still had benefits from this treatment approach after 6 six years.

Drugs used when your thyroid is underactive:

- Synthetic T4 or Levothyroxine (L-Thyroxine). Often, this is the only hormone replacement, and the conversion to the active form of thyroid hormone is assumed. Some common trade names are Levothyroxine, Synthroid, Euthyrox, Levoxyl and Oroxine.
- Synthetic T3 or Liothyronine. A manufactured version of T3 hormone. In the case symptoms remain with T4 replacement only, T3 can be used as an add-on. Doctors may be unwilling to prescribe

T3, but women who get to try it may feel persisting symptoms lift.

- Synthetic T4 and T3 combined. Compounded hormones in one pill.
- Natural dessicated thyroid. Drugs that are derived from thyroid glands of pigs and standardized to a fixed T4 to T3-ratio, called Natural Dessicated Thyroid or NDT. NDT also contain T1 and T2, hormones naturally made by the thyroid, and that may have physiological effects. Many women feel the natural hormones work better for them. The

drawback is that sometimes the concentrations of hormones in NDT do not match the prescription.

Relapses happen

Now, you may experience a relapse a while after a successful antithyroid treatment. It happen right after antithyroid medication is lifted or it can take years for the disease to reappear. Women often experience that the relapse is triggered by a traumatic event such as the death of a loved one or an accident. Many women then go back on antithyroid drugs and others choose radioactive iodine therapy or surgery of the thyroid gland. The radioiodine option means using radioactive iodine that is targeted towards the thyroid gland, is taken up by it, and the irradiation destroys it from within. This treatment has some common side effects such as lower quality of life and an increased risk of ophthalmopathy. Surgery means a removal of the thyroid gland. Both radioiodine and surgery mean that you become hypothyroid and will need to use hormonal replacement therapy for the rest of your life.

Sometimes, radioiodine or surgery are suggested to women as a first line of treatment in Graves', in that case many who would have healed from their autoimmunity are robbed of a thyroid that would function just fine in the future. All the immune system and thyroid needed was some time to calm down, and then hormonal balance would have been restored.

It can be made to seem so easy, remove the organ and then supplement with the missing hormones. Done. But for many women, hormonal replacement therapy is not all roses and sunshine, and leaves them suffering from hypothyroid symptoms instead. Hormonal therapy can be difficult to adjust and surveys show that most women on thyroid hormonal therapy still have at least one lingering symptom. Doctors may have their own idea about what is best for you, but it is your body, and you are not obligated to remove an organ just because a health care professional says so. Find another doctor to work with, someone willing to allow time for your thyroid to heal itself. For many women, that happens when treatment with antithyroid drugs is applied correctly. Even though chances are lower to go into remission if you relapse after a first successful round of antithyroids, there are women who have done so. Others continue to lean on antithyroids instead of radioiodine or surgery, even though their disease reappears every few years.

There is also opportunity in adjusting your lifestyle in such a way that your chances of becoming cured of the disease may increase. That is what "Part three – Your roadmap to healing" of this book is all about.

Thyroid storm not common but feared

One of the most feared consequences of Graves' disease is the thyroid storm. It is rare and develops with untreated hyperthyroidism, or when there is a concurrent infection. Usually, those who get thyroid storm will have one of the following triggers:

- Trauma
- Surgery
- Severe emotional distress
- Stroke
- Diabetic ketoacidosis
- Congestive heart failure
- Pulmonary embolism

The symptoms resemble hyperthyroidism but are more severe, sudden and extreme. You may have thyroid storm if you experience:

- Racing heart rate (tachycardia) that exceeds 140 beats per minute, and atrial fibrillation
- High fever
- Persistent sweating
- Shaking
- Agitation
- Restlessness
- Confusion
- Diarrhea
- Unconsciousness.

You must immediately get to the emergency room if you believe that you or someone else may have thyroid storm. Alarm the emergency number of your country right away.

Graves' and pregnancy

If a woman with Graves' disease becomes pregnant, the disease can affect both the pregnancy and the health of the mother. Pregnancy may also trigger Graves' disease in some women. If you have Graves' disease and are planning to become pregnant, it's imperative that you create a pregnancy plan with your obstetrician, endocrinologist, and other necessary specialists. Many women with Graves' disease have healthy babies, and the best chance for a healthy pregnancy and delivery is early planning and coordination with a treatment team. Talk to your doctor today about prepregnancy treatment options and how you can manage Graves' disease and also protect your child during pregnancy.

Graves' disease occurs in about 1 in 1,500 women who are pregnant, and it causes roughly 80 percent of all cases of maternal hyperthyroidism. In addition, roughly 30 percent of young women with Graves' disease were pregnant in the year prior to the onset of their symptoms. Symptoms of Graves' disease typically increase during early pregnancy and decrease during later months. Graves' disease also often becomes worse during the first three months after giving birth. The symptoms of the disease are like those in other women. Graves' disease can affect pregnancy, including these complications:

- Miscarriage

- Preterm birth
- Poor fetal growth
- Fetal thyroid dysfunction
- Maternal heart failure
- Preeclampsia (high blood pressure)
- Infertility in women and men (if the disease goes untreated).

More about the thyroid gland and the stress response

When the thyroid hormones are in balance, they are a supplement to our well-being. They deliver even energy levels and good mental health. They are also part of our adaptation to the stresses of the environment. The thyroid hormone, together with adrenaline, noradrenaline and cortisol - all of which are secreted by the adrenal glands - are important parts of our response to stress.

Beta-blockers, a drug you probably got when you were just diagnosed, reveal more about the role of the thyroid gland in the body. Beta-blockers prevent the stress hormones adrenaline and noradrenaline from affecting the cells. Many of the troublesome effects of hyperthyroidism are mediated by these. It causes the cells to increase metabolism, but it also gives us palpitations, anxiety, sweating, diarrhea, sleep problems and more. In fact, thyroid hormone makes cells more sensitive to adrenaline by giving them more receptors for the stress hormone.

Adrenaline and noradrenaline help to create the physical and mental reactions to stress. Adrenaline and noradrenaline have rapid and immediate effects in the body. In response to stress, they can be secreted from the adrenal glands in seconds and affect heart rate, energy expenditure, and prepare us for fight or flight. For example, your beating heart distributes more blood to muscles at the expense of the internal organs.

Cortisol. The task of cortisol is to be a survival hormone and free up resources to meet the immediate external threats we face. Immune system, muscle building and sleep are examples of functions that are put on hold by cortisol. Thyroid hormones make the adrenals secrete more cortisol to the point that they can become exhausted.

Three things to remember about T3

T3 is mostly known as a hormone for energy and metabolism. Yes, those are some of the primary functions, but it has far more widespread effects on our physiology. Along the book, you will be presented to more sides of this hormone and then it will be useful to remember these points about T3:

- T3 is a stress hormone. The close ties to adrenaline and cortisol make it one of our most important players in long-term regulation of adaptation to stress. When T3 goes up, so does adrenaline and cortisol.
- T3 is pro-inflammatory. Because of its connections to adrenaline, increases in T3 will cause more pro-inflammatory mediators to circulate in your body.

- T3 is vital for brain health. T3 needs to be in balance for us to feel good mentally. Too much and we become stressed out, forgetful and depressed. Too little and the result is the same. T3 needs to be in the optimal range for our social and cognitive functions to be online.

You will learn more about this and if any of these areas currently are out of balance for you – fear not. Bringing balance to the force is what part three of the book is all about.

CHAPTER 3
IMMUNE SYSTEM OUT OF BALANCE

Emma's story: I had several relapses

"I was diagnosed with Graves' when I was 16 years old. I had then felt bad for a while because it took time before I got the correct diagnosis. I lost weight and had difficulty sleeping. I noticed that something was wrong as I suddenly could not run during basketball practice without collapsing. I had a resting pulse rate at over 100 beats per minute.

When I received my diagnosis, I began taking hormonal replacement and a medication that would lower my heart rate, beta blockers. After a while, my body functioned as usual again, and I could return to training and live as I did before.

After taking medication for about 2,5 years, I stopped my treatment. There was about a 50 percent risk that I would get my Graves' back. After 2 to 3 years, it happened. It was discovered earlier this time, and I just needed to take a lower dose of medicine, this time block and replace. After about 2 years of medication, I tried again to stop the medication and hoped to avoid relapse of Graves'. I had been informed that the odds were worse this time, but I had a "mild" relapse, so there was a chance that I would be able to reverse it.

This time I once again managed for about 2 years before my Graves' came back. I experienced this relapse as more difficult as I got more mental symptoms than physical ones. I was very sensitive and had mood swings. I felt tears welling up in situations that usually did not affect me so much.

With this third relapse, I was told that I would have to have surgery to remove my thyroid gland. The odds of getting well with medication were slim now.

I had read about many people who felt bad after having surgery on their thyroid gland, that they did not get the help they needed to adjust the medicine, and reach an excellent quality of life.

My mother has had hypothyroidism for many years and in recent years she has struggled to find a doctor who will help her fully.

This made me choose medication once again. I knew that the medicine quickly restored my mood and thus I wanted to do everything to avoid surgery on my thyroid gland. My doctor agreed and together with my recent relapses being mild, we jointly concluded that this was the right decision.

As before, I managed about 2 years after finishing medication before my Graves' returned.

Now the decision was made that I would have surgery to remove my thyroid gland. Because of allergies and thus extra risks of complications, we concluded that I would have my operation at a university hospital and therefore the waiting time was longer.

While waiting for surgery, I once again took block and replace, and when it was my turn to have surgery, it turned out that all my values were normal again. Now it did not feel right to do a surgical procedure when my body was feeling well. Removing a functioning organ is not a simple decision. I did not expect to end up in this situation.

I cancelled my surgery and stopped taking medication. This time I also changed my diet to reduce inflammation in the body as inflammation can trigger Graves'.

Six months later, I got my Graves' back. This time I felt terrible and had to take sick leave from work as I neither had the energy nor could cope with the stress. Even at home I was affected. I did not want to hang out with people, and the energy for training no longer existed. We raised, lowered and raised the medicine again and in the end, I felt better but somehow I feel like the disease has made its mark on my body and my mind.

It has been five months since I had surgery to remove my thyroid gland. Today I feel better. I tried to avoid having surgery on my thyroid gland, but finally there were few other options left for me. I hope that I will feel good and that I will be listened to and get the help I need if there comes a day when I do not feel so well on my hormone replacement treatment.

I do not regret that I tried medication as many times as I did. But I wish I had learned about the impact of lifestyle earlier. Maybe it would have helped me if I had changed my diet already the first time I was diagnosed with Graves'."

*

Autoimmunity is all too common

"An ounce of prevention is worth a pound of cure"
Benjamin Franklin

At the University of Amsterdam, a study is underway with women called "Amsterdam autoimmune thyroid disease cohort". The purpose of it is to find out how we can know who is at risk of suffering from our most common thyroid diseases. The women are healthy when they join the study but have relatives with autoimmune thyroid disease. The researchers follow the women to see in which of them disease breaks out. 1000 women between the ages of 18 and 65 are taking part to help us get answers to important questions about thyroid disease. The study approach has been chosen precisely because it is well known that we who suffer have a heredity for it, but also because many environmental factors come into play. Today we already know a lot about why we get sick, including several things you can influence yourself.

For a long time, autoimmunity was considered impossible, that the body was far too wise for such self-destructive behaviour. In fact, many people have an autoimmune disease, and the healthcare costs for them are staggering. They are becoming more and more common, which is mainly believed to have to do with how we live - our lifestyle and the surrounding environment.

Your immune system

The immune system is often compared to an army that fights battles against foreign substances and organisms. The immune system originates from the bone marrow and comprises several types of cells, each with unique functions. Some parts of the immune system can direct attacks that are tailored to the intruder. This tailored type is also called acquired immunity and plays the greatest role for autoimmunity. It is a difficult balancing act the immune system must perform every day. Not only does it have to keep intruders out, it also has to recognize and clean up aged and damaged cells. The immune system can also neutralise cancer cells. Finally, it must recognize which of the cells that is its own, healthy tissue and leave it. Too often this goes wrong and an attack on one's own cells begins.

An immune response, when for example bacteria enter the body, is controlled by the white blood cells. They use their messenger mediators cytokines and hormones to target so-called antigens - foreign proteins on the intruder's surface. These foreign proteins trigger the attack from the immune system. The most important types of white blood cells in autoimmunity can be of T-cell or B-cell type. The T cells are messengers and can kill cells, while the B-cells form antibodies that flag a cell to be destroyed. Each B-cell can only make one type of antibody. TRAb is the distinctive antibody for Graves'. B-cells specialized in forming TRAb receive signals to increase in number, activate and form antibodies. When the antibodies are attached to the TSH receptor, the thyroid gland interprets that it has been stimulated by TSH and produces more hormone.

Theories about causes of autoimmune disease

Risk factors for Graves', and all autoimmune diseases can be divided into congenital, genetic and environmental factors. You cannot influence how old you are, but you have a greater influence on whether or not you are a smoker.

Evidence of how important the environmental factors are for the onset of autoimmune disease is seen if we look at how common they are in different parts of the world. They are most common in the West and less common in Asia, for example. When families move to Europe or the United States from countries where autoimmune diseases are less common, something interesting happens. The parents in the family still have the same lower risk of developing autoimmune disease, but the risk for their children increases. Same genes, different environment. This gives hope. By affecting your environment, you can also affect your health. That the environment plays a role is clear, but today there is no uniform answer why autoimmune disease arises. There are several ideas, which partly overlap, about why our bodies attack themselves:

The hygiene hypothesis. Our environment is often too sterile, say those who advocate the hygiene hypothesis. We live cleaner today than what is good for us. Our immune system needs a certain amount of external stimulation in the form of bacteria and the right kind of dirt to stay fit and react to the right things. Both allergies and autoimmunity are said to arise from this cause.

Functional medicine hypothesis. Functional medicine is an approach to medicine that comes from the United States. It is above all a way of looking at the causes and treatment of our common diseases. The medicine of why - functional medicine - means that diagnoses do not tell us anything. The names we give diseases are useful for choosing drugs, but not for finding the actual root cause or starting a healing process. Two people can have Graves' for different reasons. One person has high inflammatory markers and a stressful life, while another has infection and is a smoker. If we take the time to ask why these people got Graves', the answer to how we should behave to calm the immune system can become clearer. By thinking about why someone has developed symptoms of ill health, we find answers, often in the form of lifestyle measures to create health and an excellent quality of life.

Functional medicine has adopted a model from researcher Alessio Fasano for the emergence of autoimmunity, which describes that three things must happen simultaneously:

- A genetic sensitivity.
- Increased intestinal permeability, often called leaky gut. Substances, pieces of bacteria and other things we have in the intestine that are usually too large to get through the intestinal lining enter the body and create a reaction in the immune system. An immune system that is constantly irritated increases the risk of attacking one's own tissue. It is also possible that proteins that leaks through are like one of the body's own proteins - that is how molecular mimicry arises.
- A trigger. For example, stress, infection or low vitamin D levels.

The role of epigenetics. You might have heard: "Genes load the gun, environment pulls the trigger". The numbers vary depending on the source, but up to 30 percent of your health is affected by your genes, and the remaining at least 70 percent depends on your lifestyle and environment and not the genes themselves. This means it matters more how we live than what genes you have. The word epigenetics roughly means "above the genes". This means that molecules can be attached to the genes to make the specific gene more active or less active. An epigenetic change can prevent the reading of a gene and then no, or fewer, products are formed from it. Imagine that the book you want to read has a padlock on it you do not have the key to. Then it will be impossible for you to use the information in there, even if you hold the book in your hand. It is the same in the cell. But the cell can also put a flag on the gene that says "look here, come here and read me!" Now, more products are formed, sometimes favourable for us and in other cases bad for us. Many diseases are associated with epigenetic changes and Graves' is no exception. This means a lot for you who suspect that you have an increased risk of, for example, autoimmunity, perhaps because many relatives have been affected. With the help of your lifestyle, you can reduce your risk of getting ill.

The microbiome and autoimmune disease. That our gut, or rather the microbes in it, are crucial to our health has had a major impact. You have a unique bacterial composition, a "fingerprint" for the microbes in your gut - who they are and how many. The fingerprint can well show your health status and tell you whether you are healthy or sick. Sometimes even what disease you have. To a large extent, the focus is on the enormous opportunities this gives us in the form of affecting our gut flora to promote a healthy environment in the intestine and subsequently the entire body. The immune system resides mostly in the intestine, because the intestine is technically the outside of the body and thus in need of strict monitoring.

Risk factors associated with Graves' disease

The chance that you who are reading this are a woman, age 30 and upwards, have relatives with autoimmune diseases and at the time of diagnosis recently experienced a negative life event is significant. These are the characteristics of the most common Graves' patient.

Congenital risk factors for getting Graves':

- Women are affected five times more often by Graves' - especially when they have recently given birth or are experiencing other hormonal fluctuations such as menopause.
- Age, most commonly between 30 and 50
- Genetics.

Environmental factors:

- Smoking doubles the risk of Graves'
- Infections with coxsackie virus, Yersinia enterocolitica, Borrelia burgdorferi, Helicobacter pylori, hepatitis C and retroviruses (HTLV-1, HFV, HIV and SV40)
- Stress, usually in the form of major negative life events
- Vitamin D deficiency
- Increased inflammation markers
- Some medicines, Interferon- α, alemtuzumab
- Endocrine disrupting chemicals and heavy metals
- Altered intestinal flora.

Risk factors associated with Graves' ophthalmopathy

The causes of Graves' ophthalmopathy are not clear. It is linked to Graves', but you can get it even with balanced thyroid hormones. It can develop in just one eye and can appear several years after hyperthyroidism. All this suggests that ophthalmopathy is multifactorial, not just due to one cause.
Some established risk factors are:

- Age, older people have a higher risk of ophthalmopathy
- Smoking triples the risk of ophthalmopathy and increases the risk that it will worsen - the risk is proportional to the number of cigarettes smoked per day
- Radiation with radioactive iodine
- Selenium deficiency
- Fluctuations in thyroid hormone values
- High total and LDL cholesterol.

More about the risk factors

Female gender. Women are significantly more likely than men to suffer from autoimmune diseases and Graves' in particular. It is especially common for disease to develop during sex hormone fluctuations such as after giving birth or menopause. We still do not know exactly why women are more affected than men. Women's immune systems are more aggressive than men's, and it must be able to tolerate carrying a fetus - a foreign organism.

Genetics. Genetics is an important cause of Graves' disease and there are several variants of genes linked to the disease. For example, there are molecules on cells that are used to present pieces of proteins. These are then "read" by immune cells to determine if a cell is a friend or an enemy. With a certain presenter gene, the thyroid proteins are more likely to be mistaken as harmful, and the immune system triggers a reaction against the thyroid gland.

Smoking. A common contributing cause of several autoimmune diseases. It is not yet clear exactly how smoking causes an increased risk of getting sick, probably because it contributes to inflammation.

Infections. Infections involve a revved up immune system. There are several theories why certain infections are more common in patients with autoimmune diseases. One of them is molecular mimicry, proteins in viruses or bacteria are like our own. If the infection does not resolve, the attack is maintained. But even if the infection is dormant or has healed, the immune system can continue to attack the thyroid gland in the belief that it is working to get rid of an infection. An infection also paves the way for autoimmunity by circulating higher levels of pro-inflammatory mediators in the body and irritating the immune system.

Stress in the form of negative life events. Many of us with Graves' have a story to tell about an event just before we got sick. It may be the death of a dear one, a divorce or other things that completely shake up our world. Perhaps we never had time to mourn before the disease broke out.

When over 200 patients recently diagnosed with Graves', answered questions about their health, they reported more negative life events in the last 12 months. Other types of hyperthyroidism such as toxic multinodular adenoma do not have this connection.

Stress and the immune system are linked. The research area of psychoneuroimmunology wants to explain to us exactly what the connections between the nervous system (stress), the immune system, and our hormones look like. A simple model of how they interact is the effect of cortisol on the immune system. The hormone is secreted during various types of stress and has a powerful effect on the immune system. In the short term, this is not a problem, but when cortisol levels are high in the long term, the immune system weakens. This is then thought to lead to various types of disease, including autoimmunity.

Vitamin D deficiency. Low levels of Vitamin D increase the risk of Graves', but it is still unclear what role the vitamin has in the disease.

Inflammation. In inflammation and autoimmune disease, it is difficult to know what came first, the chicken or the egg. The disease can increase inflammation in the body, at the same time it is known that chronic low-grade inflammation lays the foundation for autoimmune diseases to appear. Graves' patients have also been found to have higher levels of chronic low-grade inflammation. The TRAb antibodies can increase inflammation inside the thyroid through increased activity in the gland. They can also lead to increased cell death, and dead cells irritate the immune system. Both can create and maintain Graves'. There are also indications that hormonal problems such as polycystic ovary syndrome (PCOS) may contribute to the development of Graves'. Women with PCOS have increased levels of TRAb and an increased risk of being diagnosed with Graves'. PCOS means a disturbed metabolism where female hormones end up out of balance and chronic low-grade inflammation. The researchers believe that it is these factors that contribute to the increased risk for Graves' in PCOS.

Endocrine disruptors and heavy metals. Every day we are exposed to chemicals through food, cleaning products, in our profession, via plastic, make-up and more. Endocrine disruptors mainly affect estrogen but also thyroid hormones. According to the WHO, such substances may influence the risk of developing autoimmune disease.

Altered intestinal flora. Studies show that the intestinal flora is altered in Graves'. It is less species-rich, which is negative as we want it to be more like a rainforest and contain many species. In addition, the number of certain bacteria is greater or fewer than normal. The changes seen are not uncommon, they appear repeatedly when the intestinal flora is measured in patients with diseases such as multiple sclerosis, asthma, cancer and more. The researchers point out the lack of bifidobacteria and lactobacilli as potentially negative. These types of bacteria are linked to good health.

Research has also predicted the levels of TRAb in the blood of patients by looking at the composition of the intestinal flora.

Risk factor or root cause? The actual reasons of your symptoms revealed

According to the father of functional medicine, Dr Jeffrey Bland, we are in a "disease delusion". We are led to believe that the only way to manage chronic diseases such as diabetes, heart disease, osteoporosis, arthritis, and dementia is to manage is by pills and temporary remedies. To dissolve symptoms of chronic disease we must, according to Dr Bland, get skilled at "identifying, preventing, and addressing their underlying causes". Functional medicine practitioners ask why you got ill, the look for the root causes of disease, so they can find a plan that is personalized for you. They put you at the centre and look at you as a whole, your physical, mental, emotional and spiritual wellbeing. You are also treated as a whole, all the organs and their functioning are tied together. If two people have Graves', their root causes of getting ill needs to be revealed. They also need to be seen as individuals with the ability to self-heal. You will have to do your part, but the upside is that you regain power of your health and well-being.

But what can underlie causes of chronic disease and Graves' in particular? Some commonly mentioned root causes of disease are:

- Stress, emotional and mental
- Food insensitivities
- Gut Imbalances
- Nutritional deficiencies
- Toxins
- Infections.

Look again at the risk factors in Graves' and you see that many of them match one of these root causes. But what exactly is the difference between a root cause and a risk factor? Here is an example: For many of us, Graves' is caused by the root cause inflammation. Anything increasing the individual's exposure or susceptibility to inflammatory mediators is then a risk factor.

This may be age - you have more inflammation as you get older, smoking, stress or genetics. The reason we must look for the root causes and dig them out is because this may resolve autoimmunity and any lingering symptoms. These root causes, if left in the ground, will cause imbalances unique to each person. In one person with Graves' maybe the nervous system takes the biggest hit and in another the skeleton. The flip side of the coin is that these are an opportunity for finding the root causes of healing. In part three you will self-test what root causes of healing are most important for you to focus on.

Hedvig's story: The power of self-healing

"Sometimes positive stories are needed. And I really think mine has been so far.

I was diagnosed in March 2018. I was feeling terrible then, with all the symptoms you can have except weight loss. Because of my mood, my partner and I broke up. He could not bear me feeling so bad. As soon as I began treatment, my life changed. I found the right dose of block and replace and after only six months on the medicine, my values were good and remained so throughout the treatment. Now in May 2020 I have been without medicine for a month and had my first follow-up today. My hormone levels are perfect. And I feel great! And have been doing so for 1,5 years now. I am so grateful for all the help I received and how well it went.

There are many of you out there who are having a hard time and I suffer with you. I remember so well what it was like before the diagnosis. But for those of you who are new to the disease -

there is hope. Everything does not have to be pitch black. I hope more people get the same "easy" course that I got."

*

How common is it to be cured from Graves'?

The definition of being cured by Graves', according to researchers at the University of Amsterdam, could be: Stable TSH, levels of free T4 and T3 within normal values and that the person is not treated with thyroid medication. The absence of antibodies to the thyroid gland could be added to the definition.

In many countries, the standard treatment is the block and replace. Research at several European hospitals shows that if 100 women are diagnosed with Graves' and treated by block and replace, 40 of them will have normal thyroid values without medical treatment for thyroid disease eight years later. We know nothing about what their antibodies look like, other than that they can be considered cured.

50 of the 100 women will have had radioiodine or surgery.

The last 10 women have normal thyroid values with the help of hormone replacement.

Although the last two groups may very well feel fully recovered from the disease, they have hypothyroidism, an underactive thyroid gland.

What does it really matter if you are declared cured or not?

In quality of life, the often impaired in Graves', it can play a role. Freedom from chronic illness is associated with a higher quality of life than if you suffer from an autoimmune disease, cardiovascular disease, or mental illness. There are individual differences and those declared cured may have a poorer quality of life than those who are not.

One of the most common reasons patients themselves state that they do not feel recovered from Graves' is, as we have seen before, concerns about living with a lifelong illness where there is a risk that the disease will return.

Factors in Graves' that speak for or against a recovery

During treatment with medication, the levels of TRAb often decrease and when you remove the medication after a while, a large proportion have gotten rid of the symptoms. For others, the levels of antibodies may rise again, even if they have been low during treatment. The risk of relapse decreases, after which time passes. Most relapse within 1 year, the prognosis to avoid relapse after 4 years is good.

Some believe that the drugs that block hormone production given in Graves' help the body return to normal thyroid levels, and that allows the immune system to calm down again. Others believe that it is the antithyroid drugs themselves given in Graves' that directly affect the immune system:

- They have an immunosuppressive effect and reduce TRAb in your blood

- Immune cells in the thyroid associated with autoimmunity die of the process called programmed cell death
- Increases the number of suppressing T-cells which calms the immune system,
- Lower numbers of overactive T-helper cells.

This facilitates achievement of remission of Graves' disease. PTU may also act in the peripheral tissues by inhibiting conversion of thyroxine to triiodothyronine. Metronidazole may also act as an antioxidant in the thyroid. Treatment with blocking drugs for a longer time than usual is more common today and may also lead to a greater proportion of patients who get cured.

Every disease has a so-called natural course. That means how the disease develops if it is not treated. Not much is known about Graves' natural course, but a research article states that given that many of us relapse, a smaller proportion would only have one bout of hyperthyroidism. Others may - if they do not stop the autoimmune process - expect new episodes of hyperthyroidism and relapse.

Besides the effect of treatment on the risk of recurrence, we also need to consider the clinical picture at the time of diagnosis. In studies, researchers have developed a checklist to determine who has a better chance of being declared healthy and who may relapse. Just remember: you are an individual and have a chance to get well no matter what your circumstances say. Statistics tell us about the average outcome of all the sick, but you are an individual and your recovery is not out of reach even if you have things that speak against. Also, if you change the lifestyle factors that are root causes of disease, which we will discuss in the book, you may change your conditions completely. Factors in illness that increase your chances of being cured:

- Female gender, men have a higher risk of relapse.
- One or fewer relatives with Graves'.
- TSH value above 0.4.
- TPO antibodies below 10,000.
- fT4 under 40.
- No occurrence of TRAb, the lower the better for your chances of recovery.
- Thyrotropin binding inhibitory immunoglobulins (TBII) below 20.
- Becoming ill after the age of 40, at the same time older age, means a greater risk of developing ophthalmopathy.
- The size of the goiter according to the WHO classification is less than Grade II.
- Have not had hyperthyroidism for over 4 months.
- No presence of genes that increase the risk of Graves'.
- No symptoms of Graves' ophthalmopathy, and if they occur, they are less severe.
- No stress in the form of negative life events or in everyday life.

Spotlight on: Other autoimmune diseases in Graves'

When we do not feel well despite treatment for hyperthyroidism, it is sometimes because we have another autoimmune diagnosis. Mainly Hashimoto's thyroiditis but also:

- Atrophic gastritis (B12 deficiency)
- Addison's disease
- Diabetes type-1,
- Gluten intolerance (celiac disease),
- Vitiligo
- Rheumatoid arthritis
- Sjögren syndrome
- Alopecia.

These are examples of autoimmune diseases that are associated with Graves' and partly have the same genetic causes. If you have an autoimmune disease, the risk of getting more autoimmune diseases increases. About 10 percent of those with Graves' have more autoimmune diseases.

Risk of developing Hashimoto's

Hypothyroidism is the most common type of thyroid disorder. The most common form of hypothyroidism is autoimmune and is called Hashimoto's thyroiditis. But why bother about that when you have Graves'? Well, you need to be aware of your increased risk of developing hypothyroidism.

Sometimes, the immune response in Graves' can cause the thyroid tissue to be destroyed, and it causes a suboptimal function, or low thyroid values. After Graves', it is also common to experience a gradual switch to Hashimoto's. Researchers believe that these diagnoses are two sides of the same coin, in part it is the same antibodies that are present even though TRAb dominates in Graves' and antibodies against thyroid peroxidase (TPO) and thyroglobulin

(TG) in Hashimoto's. These are examples of early symptoms of hypothyroidism:

- Fatigue or less physical strength
- Depression
- Difficulties concentrating
- Freezing.

Later you may have these symptoms:

- Dry skin and dry hair
- Constipation
- Weight gain
- Memory difficulties
- Slow heartbeat
- Pain in joints and muscles
- Fertility issues.

If you have had hypothyroidism for a long time without treatment, you may get a swelling on your face and your voice may become darker. If you did not get goiter because of Graves', you can now get it because of Hashimoto's. Take thyroid tests regularly, hypothyroidism often comes on slowly, unlike hyperthyroidism, which comes more suddenly.

Celiac disease is common in Graves'

There are those who argue that everyone with Graves' should also be screened for celiac disease because they often occur together. Celiac disease (also called gluten intolerance) is another common, autoimmune disease and millions of people around the world are diagnosed. There are several reasons celiac disease and thyroid disease can affect you at the same time:

- They have common genetic causes
- Both are relatively common autoimmune diseases
- One autoimmune disease increases the risk of being diagnosed with more.

Both celiac disease and hyperthyroidism affect the entire body, therefore the diseases also have common symptoms. This can be, for example, fatigue, memory problems or symptoms from the gastrointestinal tract, depression or hair loss. Celiac disease can make you absorb drugs less efficiently from the intestine, including hormonal replacement. Fluctuating hormone levels in blood tests may therefore be a sign that you have an inflammation in the gut, possibly caused by celiac disease. If you have symptoms that may show gluten intolerance, you can ask for a test. Just remember not to exclude gluten before doing the test as the risk then is that it is not possible to measure antibodies.

When hormone replacement treatment is not enough

Dear reader, please note: Most Graves' patients switch to hypothyroidism. During your block and replace, and when you have been treated with radioiodine or surgery, you practically have hypothyroidism. In addition, many of us eventually get Hashimoto's thyroiditis. Hypothyroidism is when your thyroid gland alone does not produce enough hormone for your needs. As for us with Graves', many with hypothyroidism experience reduced quality of life. 20 percent are not recovered despite treatment, and 60 percent have at least some symptoms with an impact on their daily lives. Several of the patients in long-term studies of Graves' patients tell that they are not happy with their hormone replacement therapy. It is the treatment you receive instead of your thyroid's own hormones, usually synthetic T4 and patients sometimes point to that it may be the reason they do not feel recovered. Many believe that synthetic T4 is not enough for everyone and some get supplementation of T3. A smaller proportion receive Natural Dessicated Thyroid (NDT), which is dried porcine thyroid. A potential problem with T4 in tablet form is that it assumes its conversion to the active T3 in the body. But people treated with T4 have a lower ratio of T3 to T4 than healthy people. A low T3 ratio shows that we are not converting T4 to T3. Then we cannot take advantage of the active hormone we need to feel good. Graves' patients who have undergone radioiodine treatment and are treated with T4 have a lower T3: T4 ratio than patients only treated with antithyroid (the drugs that reduce the thyroid glands' hormone production). Some common reasons T4 is not converted to T3: chronic low-grade inflammation, high cortisol levels, nutritional deficiencies, genetic variants of enzymes responsible for the conversion of T4 or imbalances in the intestinal flora. If you suspect that your replacement therapy is a cause of your symptoms, talk to your doctor about how to adjust the treatment.

Some excellent resources for learning more about hypothyroidism, please see the books of Dr Amy Myers, Izabella Wentz and Dr Aviva Romm.

Sometimes the thyroid gland takes the blame for all the symptoms and all our experience of ill health. Keep an open mind for other reasons you are not feeling well.

PART TWO - BODY OUT OF BALANCE

The body is a multifaceted and complex organism, where everything is connected. Therefore, we cannot really take one aspect of health out of context. A human being is a functioning whole - when we look closer, there is no division. It does not matter if we are talking about the interaction between body and mind or how the different physiological systems work together. By a physiological system is meant, for example, the nervous system, the endocrine system or the musculoskeletal system.

Part two describes common health problems in connection with Graves'. Soon you notice that there are a lot of points of contact between them. Therefore, remember that your body functions as a whole - not separate systems.

My story: From healthy to feeling well

In 2017, I was cured but did not feel well. Those are not the same thing as I have learned. I had perfect hormone values in my blood and was cured but felt awful. I still experienced a lot of fatigue and was sensitive to stress. My energy levels were low. I had to resign from freelance assignments that I really enjoyed very much, slept whenever I got the chance, did as little as possible in all areas of my life. I had only two gears. I either felt revved up, burning all reserves. Or exhausted, my body weighed a ton, and I struggled through my days. My family also had to suffer for how I felt. I remember one night when I was putting the kids to bed. Then my five-year-old son took my face in his hands and said: "I feel so sorry for you who cannot come with us on all the fun things we do."

That stress was lingering on after the disease was clear to me, and I searched for a solution. Tried supplements, sleeping more, more exercise - less exercise, more carbohydrates - fewer carbohydrates. Despite my efforts, I did not reach my goal of more energy, instead the spiral went downwards. I got more and more tired and less and less able to do things in my daily life. One day when I was out for a walk, I listened to a podcast and learned about the effects of meditation on the brain.

After 8 weeks of meditation, 40 minutes a day, subjects in one study had experienced measurable changes in several areas of the brain. I had been curious about meditation before, but this was exactly what I needed to hear. Real measurable effects on the brain - I decided right away that I would try. I gave it 30 days and thought to meditate 40 minutes every day - it did not have to be all in one go, but 10 minutes here and 20 there was approved. At first, I had no thoughts that meditation would solve my remaining health challenges.

When I started meditating that day, I had no high expectations at all, I thought it sounded good that the brain could change for the better. It was a joyful surprise when things started happening. During the first few weeks, I finally found a pause button for my stress. Meditation had become a tool to use when I needed to calm down. Invaluable. When the 30 days had passed, I was hooked and continued to meditate every day. Then it took maybe 3 months before I started getting more results, and I did not expect them either. I was just happy and satisfied to break my stress. Now, the spiral turned and become positive. From having endured less and less, I could do more and more. Today I can come along for all the fun things my family do.

Interview with Kerstin Brismar, Professor and specialist in endocrinology: Lifestyle is important in thyroid disease

Kerstin Brismar is a professor at the Department of Molecular Medicine and Surgery, a specialist in endocrinology and diabetology. She has treated many patients with Graves', is the author of hundreds of research studies, and is interested in the impact of lifestyle on our health. Kerstin Brismar pointed out in a debate article from 2018:

“Many thyroid patients continue to feel unwell despite treatment. We must invest in research of personalized care for these patients.”

Kerstin Brismar believes that lifestyle is important and always asks her patients how they live.

"With Graves’, stress is a major factor to consider, as a severe stress often can trigger the disease. Before we had access to today's treatment options, patients had to lie in a quiet, room without stimuli. We also gave beta blockers that reduced symptoms. The disease could heal by itself but sometimes it took a long time.”

Kerstin says that in Graves’, it is the same lifestyle factors that come into play as in other diseases.

"Good sleep strengthens our immune system, diet is important, also physical activity. These affect our mood. But in Graves’ you do not have the same strength or condition. Then you cannot tell the patient to exercise immediately, but it is important later on. With diet, some people become very hungry and may not make the best dietary choices but eat processed food. Unfortunately, there are few studies that show how diet affects autoimmune processes. There are some studies that show that diet can affect inflammation in the body, if we eat better it decreases. When the disease is active, try to be kind to the body and eat nutritious food, but currently there is no science behind it.”

Lifestyle changes should be a collaboration

During lifestyle changes, both doctor and patient can contribute to successful implementation. They have different roles, but a collaboration is important for the result.

"The doctor's task is to inform about what they know scientifically and from their experience. I usually give practical advice to follow. I inform about different lifestyle factors and then the patient can tell me what they want to change. Is it diet, sleep, physical activity, or stress management? If you do everything at once usually nothing sticks. It is good to give a basic knowledge of all the lifestyle factors but begin with one of them. I have seen that gives a ripple effect but the first time it was quantified was when we did a 5: 2 study. When the participants started eating less, other things also improved. Sleep became better, they were more cheerful, moved more, several factors were affected. The patient must be motivated to do at least something. Many are not. They do not have the strength to try. In the beginning, it can be a sacrifice to change habits. But there are also those who are very motivated and when they get the right tools, they change their lifestyle."

The role of lifestyle in recovery

With Graves', there is a chance to be cured, but the question is whether lifestyle can be a factor in recovery. There are many patient stories, but there are still no major studies showing the connection.

"We do not know if lifestyle matters in being cured from Graves'. A researcher in the Netherlands is looking at relapses and what is causing them. But theoretically we know that stress is a key factor. Not taking care of your health, by not doing what you know is the best for your health can create anxiety and stress symptoms. Therefore, I can imagine that it could help if you change your lifestyle. It may not apply to everyone."

In Graves', there is a risk that autoimmunity will slip into Hashimoto's. Kerstin Brismar has met several such patients:

"Some Graves' patients get what we call a "hashicosis". An autoimmune process creates an inflammation that knocks out the thyroid gland partially or completely. It can initially present as Graves' with antibodies to TSH. Several types of antibodies against the thyroid gland are present at diagnosis and then you can suspect that this patient will get a hypothyroidism later. You can see this early on. I always measure all the antibodies that are possible, and if I see several of them, I follow my patients. Sometimes the patient recovers quickly from Graves' and instead switches to hypothyroidism."

Remaining symptoms may be because of hypothyroidism and Kerstin Brismar provides lifestyle advice that increases the levels of active T3:

• Reduce all fast carbs (avoid soft drinks, juices, everything with extra added sugar, diet based on white flour, white rice, minimize bread)

• Avoid processed foods, also semi-finished products with many additives

• Do not eat between meals

- Eat or drink no calories in the evening or during the night. 12 to 14 hours of daily fasting from evening to morning is recommended.
- Walking 30 minutes outside (or 15 x 2) every day and in addition 30 minutes outside with more intense physical activity three times per week is an excellent solution.
- Methods for stress management and recovery are recommended, 7 to 8 hours of good sleep is important.

CHAPTER 4
INFLAMMATION AS A ROOT CAUSE

There are three reasons inflammation is especially important to know for Graves' patients.

- An inflammation inside the thyroid gland and/or in the body can trigger autoimmunity.
- Once the autoimmune disease is up and running, the activated immune system creates further chronic low-grade inflammation in your body.
- The disease finally contributes to inflammation because of the pro-inflammatory effect of T3.

Inflammation is really something useful. We need it for our survival, and it occurs when the immune system is activated for various reasons. For example, when you become infected with a virus or injure yourself. Inflammation is a natural part of our defence. The inflammation is there to keep intruders out and heal our wounds by stimulating growth of new tissue and facilitating the transport of oxygen and nutrients to the site of injury. The process called acute inflammation is a good thing when you need it.

A more harmful type of inflammation is the chronic low-grade type. Instead of the immune system making a short effort, it more or less constantly sends out inflammatory mediators that circulate in your body. Inflammatory mediators are harmful to cells and tissues in the long run. These pro-inflammatory mediators that fight bacteria or viruses that have caused infection now turn on our own cells. When they are affected by chronic inflammation, this can cause many symptoms because the tissues do not thrive in an environment that was supposed to be used in an emergency for a limited amount of time. Normal inflammation:

- Healing and repairing wounds and injuries
- When meeting good bacteria in the gut
- Infection from less good bacteria.

Harmful inflammation:

- Allergy
- Autoimmunity
- Chronic infection
- Low-grade inflammation caused by an inflammatory lifestyle.

Inflammation is found at the root of autoimmune disease, and inflammation increases when the immune system is active. When the immune system fights its own body in the belief that the cells are invaders, it also spits out the pro-inflammatory mediators that have been shown to have harmful effects on our health. Your lifestyle is a potentially powerful way to reduce your inflammation.

A common measure of chronic low-grade inflammation is C-reactive protein, CRP. The protein is produced in the liver in response to inflammation in the body and can be easily measured with a blood test. CRP is elevated in hyperthyroidism compared to when we have stable thyroid hormones. A small study found that people with Graves' had a CRP of on average 4. The functional medicine doctor Mark Hyman says: "Your CRP should be lower than 1. All over it is a big warning flag that you have hidden inflammation." Often, a more sensitive form of measuring CRP is used in detecting chronic low-grade inflammation: hs-CRP (highly sensitive CRP).

Inflammation at the core of disease

In connection with acute or chronic low-grade inflammation, cytokine levels in the blood rise. They activate the immune system and can make the brain understand that we are sick. Cytokines cause the so-called disease response, something we all recognize from when we are feeling sick:

- Fatigue, increased need for sleep
- Depression, anxiety or worry
- Increased pain sensitivity
- Changed appetite
- Decreased interest in social activities.

The purpose of feeling bad during acute inflammation is that we should withdraw from people when we are infected to avoid infecting others, and also because we should rest. Injuries and infections take a lot of energy f ear body to heal. With low-grade inflammation, we do not feel as bad as when we have acute inflammation for a limited time, but we feel a little bad for a long time.

There are several ways the lifestyle can contribute to inflammation. Toxic substances, food sensitivities, chronic infection, sugar, processed foods, fats such as omega-6 and trans fats, injuries and stress can all contribute to chronic inflammation. And chronic inflammation is a factor in all major diseases: autoimmunity but also cardiovascular disease, type

2 diabetes, dementia, cancer and many more. But long before you become ill, you suspect that something is wrong. Fatigue, headaches and difficulty thinking are all examples of early signs of chronic inflammation. You vaguely recognize the symptoms from the disease response, but the effect is not as dramatic. The symptoms can also come and go. We get used to not feeling up to par and may not notice how bad we feel until we get rid of the chronic inflammation. Here are some signs that you may have low-grade chronic inflammation:

- Swelling
- Fatigue, even without obvious causes
- Unexplained pains and aches
- Depression
- Brain fog
- Sore joints
- Gastrointestinal problems.

Leaky gut - cause of inflammation

The intestinal mucosa, the barrier between the intestine and the body, is only a single cell layer thick. This does not stop it from being very efficient in its job. To help strengthen the barrier and allow the cells to hook into each other, it has proteins called tight junctions. The intestine is always semi permeable and lets through nutrients and fluid that pass into the body. Increased permeability can occur when tight junctions release from each other and there is a larger gap. Causes of this can be inflammation, infection, food sensitivities or medication. Increased permeability is also called leaky gut. With leaky gut, undigested food, toxins, and parts of bacteria enter the body. These can all activate the immune system and give symptoms anywhere in the body. Common causes of leaky gut:

- Imbalance in the intestinal flora with more harmful bacteria and fewer protective good bacteria
- Stress, emotional or physical
- Gluten from wheat, rye, and barley
- Antibiotics
- Previous or ongoing infections by bacteria, viruses, Candida, or parasites
- Common prescription free painkillers such as paracetamol, acetylsalicylic acid, or ibuprofen
- Alcohol
- Environmental toxins
- Lectins are found in certain foods and can attach to the intestinal wall.

Inflammation in Graves'

Besides the chronic low-grade inflammation caused by a constantly irritated immune system, in Graves' we have additional inflammation to deal with. It comes from the activation of the stress response.

An important part of the stress response is to provide enough energy for fight or flight, that causes increased metabolism in Graves'. Oxygen, glucose and fatty acids are delivered to the cells' energy factories - the mitochondria - to form life-sustaining molecules. Normally, the mitochondria take the food we eat - or energy we have stored - and convert it into energy we can use when we take on our chores for the day. But it comes with a price. A by-product of energy production are free radicals, notorious for causing inflammation. 90 percent of the body's free radicals are formed in the mitochondria. Free radicals are signals to the immune system to increase the release of cytokines. Free radicals must be quickly neutralized by antioxidants so they do not cause too many problems. Usually, the balance is maintained between energy production on the one hand and antioxidants on the other. We get antioxidants in our diet, but we can also make them ourselves. Under certain unfortunate circumstances, the number of free radicals may be greater than the antioxidants can capture. Here we encounter a new kind of stress we may be exposed to: oxidative stress. Someone has likened oxidative stress to what happens when we cut an apple and leave it on the kitchen counter in the heat. Soon, all the antioxidants in the apple have been used up and it becomes brown from the oxidation. You know that hyperthyroidism is synonymous with high metabolism. Energy production is fast and spits out plenty of free radicals. Hyperthyroidism therefore also means increased oxidative stress.

A way to calm autoimmunity can be reducing free radicals as they can cause cells to die prematurely. Cells that die prematurely must be taken care of by immune cells that specialize in "eating up" and breaking them down. The breakdown and the undigested parts of dead cells and the increased inflammation in high cell death can trigger the part of the immune system that creates and maintains autoimmunity. Therefore, free radicals can trigger autoimmunity, but they can also maintain it.

TSH - and the antibodies to TSH in Graves' - can increase the production of antioxidants in the thyroid gland to above normal levels. This is partly because TRAb can increase cell death in the thyroid gland. The body can respond to that to some extent by increasing its production of antioxidants, but the net effect in Graves' is an oxidative stress. The effects of treatment in patients with Graves' are that the production of free radicals decreases when the levels of T3 decrease. Free radicals can also be reduced more rapidly at diagnosis with the addition of antioxidants, which is discussed in the chapter on diet.

Additional inflammation in Graves' comes from the fact that the stress response can activate the immune system. The nervous system has branches into the lymphatic system where the immune cells are located and can thus influence them to spit out pro-inflammatory mediators. For one of the most important pro-inflammatory mediators, IL-6, levels are elevated in Graves'. These decrease again with treatment, but for patients with eye disease, the elevated levels seem to remain despite normal hormone levels.

Mitochondria and inflammation

In normal cases, when many free radicals are in circulation, the mitochondria themselves take a beating. They are even the part of the cell that is primarily in the firing line for free radicals. Therefore, symptoms in Graves' could be linked to the mitochondria not functioning properly. Non-functioning mitochondria can be recognized under a microscope. They become smaller, break into pieces, and you can measure that they do not produce energy with the same efficiency. There are animal studies that show that rats with hyperthyroidism find it more difficult to recover after a heart attack if they have affected mitochondria. The mitochondria are protected by the thyroid hormones from damage. T3 also increases the formation of new mitochondria, although a reduction in mitochondrial formation has been seen in people who have ophthalmopathy and are smokers. Small studies could not show that the mitochondria in Graves' get a different appearance or that they would have reduced efficiency in their energy production. Damaged or inefficient mitochondria are discussed in many diseases, including chronic fatigue syndrome/ME, many other autoimmune diseases such as Hashimoto's and multiple sclerosis and diabetes type 2. A theory called "Cell Danger Response " mean that threats to our cells, where free radicals are counted, may impair mitochondria. Cell danger response has been measured in people with chronic fatigue in the form of changes in biochemistry. The cell and sometimes the whole human, according to the researchers in the area, go into hibernation. To wake them up again, we must remove what caused the cell danger response and convince the cell that the danger is over. If it were possible to point to affected mitochondria in Graves', it would explain symptoms such as fatigue. Today there are no clear answers, hopefully we will know with more research.

Neuroinflammation as a cause of mental illness

Inflammation can also affect the brain, so-called neuroinflammation. Just as in other organs, inflammation in the brain can be beneficial with the potential to protect and heal injuries or infections. Problems arise when we have inflammation for a long time. Besides nerve cells, there are so-called support cells in the brain protecting the nerve cells and creating an environment where they can function well. Compared with the nerve cells themselves, the support cells were long considered being passive and unimportant for our brain health. The situation has proven to be the reverse, and one type of support cell is especially central. This support cell is called microglia. Microglia are formally part of the immune system. Both unbalanced microglia and nerve cells contribute to mental illness. Prolonged and incorrect activation of microglia results in a continuous release of pro-inflammatory mediators in the brain and can contribute to Alzheimer's, Parkinson's disease and mental illnesses such as schizophrenia and bipolar disorder but also fatigue and the reduction in cognitive abilities we see with unhealthy aging. Normal levels of T3 are important for the function of microglia. Disturbed hormone levels can impair the function of this cell type, make them overactive and disrupt the brain, which can be a contributing cause of mental illness.

The brain and immune system can "talk" to each other through proinflammatory mediators. These have powerful effects on the brain. When we are sick, this is good for us, but when the inflammation is chronic and low-grade, as with autoimmunity, pro-inflammatory mediators and overactive microglia risk leading to problems with our mental health, including depression.

Spotlight on: Cardiovascular health

Cardiovascular diseases are some of our most common diseases. They are multifactorial, often caused by lifestyle. Therefore, we cannot say that Graves' alone causes cardiovascular disease, even if those who have had it have an increased risk. No one knows exactly why those who previously had Graves' even 20 years later have a higher risk of developing cardiovascular disease, but there are some ways Graves' potentially contributes.

In Graves', there is pressure on the heart and blood vessels via the part of the nervous system that increases heart rate and blood pressure. Atrial fibrillation, high blood pressure, atherosclerosis, stroke and heart failure are also common.

Oxidative stress is closely linked to cardiovascular disease and contributes to several of the most common diagnoses. The heart muscle is the most mitochondria rich tissue in the body. Coenzyme Q10 (CoQ10) is an important compound to help the mitochondria generate energy, but also acts as an antioxidant and take care of harmful by-products from the process. Convenient, because energy production is a major source of free radicals. CoQ10 is a protector of the heart, and the levels are low in Graves'. A comment from researchers who measured blood levels of CoQ10 in patients with Graves' is that equally low levels have never been measured in humans before. Q10 is produced by the cells from tyrosine, which is also the building block for thyroid hormones. With an increased need for tyrosine and higher oxidative stress, it is therefore no wonder that the levels are low in Graves'.

With treatment for hyperthyroidism, we stop the production of free radicals and calm pulse and blood pressure, but what damage has been done before that? The risk of cardiovascular disease decreases when hormone levels normalize, but 20 years after diagnosis, patients still have an increased risk of high blood pressure atherosclerosis and heart failure. The American Thyroid Association concludes that it is important for hyperthyroidism patients, even if treatment is stopped, to use their lifestyle to counteract the increased risk of cardiovascular disease. Cardiovascular health depends on low inflammation, but also on a flexible nervous system. As we will see in the chapter on the brain and nervous system, imbalances in these can also be contributing factors to impaired cardiovascular health in Graves'.

CHAPTER 5
BRAIN AND NERVOUS SYSTEM UNDER PRESSURE

Jennifer's story: I was dropped like a hot potato when there were no more drugs to give

"I was diagnosed with Graves' over six years ago but still have many symptoms such as increased sensitivity to stress, poor memory, and palpitations. My opinion is that patients should be offered to take part in the same rehabilitation that is offered to others suffering from burnout.

Even though I was diagnosed in 2014, it is likely that the disease has been there for almost 30 years. Over the years, I have performed examinations on my heart and received antidepressant medication (SSRIs), with no improvement in my symptoms. Despite blood tests for thyroid hormones, it has never been concluded that it caused the problems.

Four years ago, the problems reached a kind of peak - or rather a bottom. After several trips to the health center, where I was dismissed as suffering from a seasonal affective depression, I could barely walk, had a resting heart rate of 120 beats per minute, severe sleep problems, had lost a lot of weight and severe memory problems - but I still struggled on with work and family. My husband took me by the arm, and we went to the health center - again.

I got to see a new doctor. When he looked at me and said that he did not think the problems were in my head at all, my jaw dropped. What? Are you taking me seriously? As soon as the test results came back, including for the thyroid gland, I was immediately taken off sick and "went home and died". From there, my memory became much worse. Bank codes, children's names and names of everyday things like milk were impossible to remember.

Even today, the suites after the illness linger on and affect my life a lot. The slightest stress, strain or poor sleep makes me forget things and get physically ill with palpitations and tremors. It is a big problem in my everyday life with everything that needs to be kept track of and dealt with when you have a job and family. Everything must be written down for it to be done. If I even remember to write it down.

A period after I was finished with block and replace treatment, I was very exhausted, tired and worn out and booked a visit with my endocrinologist. Just getting in the car to go to the doctor was almost insurmountable. Once I got there, I broke down and said that I cannot take it anymore, everything was too tough. The doctor replied that it was a crisis reaction I had, that it was in my head, and wrote a referral to the counsellor. My interpretation of my body was that I suffered from stress and exhaustion.

If I could make a wish for the care of Graves' patients, it would be more support after stopping treatment with block and replace. Especially in rehabilitation of stress sensitivity. Stress management and learning to wind down are examples of things I would have liked to have access to, just like other patients who are rehabilitated after being exposed to severe stress, for example, in burnout.

Healthcare drops you like a hot potato when there are no more drugs to give. We need to get doctors to listen to their patients. We know our own bodies, and if something is not right with it."

*

The effect of the disease on mental health

"Anyone who treats a patient with hyperthyroidism understands the value of a peaceful environment and calm feelings for the treatment."
Doctor Agnes Conrad, 1934

What made you see a doctor in the first place may not have been the classic symptoms of hyperthyroidism: tremors, diarrhea, swollen and enlarged thyroid gland, weight loss, palpitations or sweating. Instead, for many, it is the change in mental well-being that makes them suspect that something is wrong. Some of the most common mental symptoms are:

- Irritation
- Anxiety
- Sleeping problems
- Anger
- Crying easily
- Easily frightened
- Lack of attention
- Poor ability to concentrate
- Memory problems.

The symptoms of hyperthyroidism can be like anxiety disorder, depression, bipolar disorder or other mental illness. This can sometimes lead to Graves' being mistaken for mental illness, which is why the right lab samples are not always taken and the correct diagnosis is delayed. If we also waited to seek help, it may have taken a long time before we received the right care.

The environment may experience that the patients in the acute phase are not themselves, that communication is difficult. Even patients can often say that they do not recognize their personality, that they want to go back to how they were before. In Graves', the brain is severely affected. The emotional parts of the brain are overactive and cause us to act more emotionally than usual, while our more analytical parts of the brain are left behind. Many of us also have cognitive problems long after we have normal thyroid levels. Up to 35 percent of all patients, even with normal thyroid hormones, say that they have an increased mental fatigue. Fatigue is also something many with Graves' state as a reason for reduced quality of life. Impairments in brain function can persist for a long time, 10 years after diagnosis, Graves' patients still perform worse on psychological tests than control groups.

Mats Holmberg, medical doctor and researcher at Sahlgrenska University Hospital in Gothenburg, has defended his dissertation on Graves' and summarizes the difficulties: "Healthcare rarely has anything to offer these patients who suffer from residual mental symptoms. It is frustrating both for the patients who are left to fend for themselves to deal with the disabling symptoms and also for the clinician whose contribution to the patient's well-being is limited to compassion".

The brain and nervous system

Your brain is an amazing creation, with the task of keeping you alive and well. It keeps track of internal factors such as oxygen level and need for sleep but also external threats to you, such as an angry dog or the edge of a cliff. To help monitor the environment, the brain has our senses (sight, hearing, touch, taste and smell) and a part of the nervous system called the autonomic nervous system. Autonomous precisely because we mostly cannot control it with our will. With the help of the autonomic nervous system, the brain can collect information about, for example, pulse and breathing, but also the occurrence of infection and inflammation and other things the brain needs to be aware of to regulate our internal environment. The brain also sends signals via the autonomic nervous system to change the internal environment when it is not promoting survival. It can be about raising blood sugar, speeding up the heart or making us fall asleep.

Parts of your brain, important in Graves'

Your brain and nervous system have several parts, some of which are more important to know in Graves' than others. We will go through them in this chapter. They are:

- Limbic system with its parts amygdala and hippocampus
- Frontal lobe
- Autonomic nervous system which is divided into two parts: sympathetic and parasympathetic nervous system
- Hypothalamic-Adrenal Axis (HPA Axis).

The limbic system

The limbic system is called the mammalian brain because it is also found in other mammals. Limbus means " edge " or " border " in Latin, and the system is on the border between newer and older parts of the brain. The limbic system helps you learn things, including what you need to be vigilant about in your environment. If you have met a nasty dog, the limbic system will remind you of it the next time you meet a dog - even if it is not the same one. This part of the brain provides access to an amazing ability - to create social bonds. That we care about each other is thanks to the limbic system. Both negative and positive emotions can be found here.

Part of the limbic system, the amygdala, are two almond-shaped nuclei in the brain and are usually described as important for emotions and motivation. It plays a crucial role when we process both positive and negative stimuli and give events their emotional significance. The amygdala captures potentially dangerous events and activates the stress response. The hippocampus is a well-known part of the limbic system, linked to many important abilities: memory, exploration, imagination, creativity, creating and maintaining social bonds, and language.

The limbic system is part of our response to stress, when we urgently need to react in a situation, the brain will redirect the activity to these of our older, more emotional parts. These parts are therefore sensitive to stress. During prolonged stress, changes occur in the system which promote survival in the moment, but we experience as negative in the long run. The amygdala has an increase in activity while the hippocampus decreases in activity. This can cause us feeling depressed, anxious, tired and downright burnt out.

Not only size matters

It may be true that if you have a large social network, you will have an easier time to find the right help when needed. But sometimes the quality, which people you have connections to, is the most important thing. The brain works in the same way. A larger hippocampus usually predicts better function, but how well the connections to other parts of the brain work also play a role. When a person has neurological or psychiatric symptoms, a connection is seen between a smaller hippocampus and poorer memory. However, the size differs when healthy controls are examined, younger people seem to have a better memory if they have a smaller hippocampus. When older people are studied, it seems to be the case that they need to have a larger hippocampus plus good connections to other parts of the brain to learn new things.

Frontal lobe

At the front of the brain you will find the frontal lobe. It is the seat of your personality, and it is this part of the brain that is said to make us human. It is one reason we humans have tall foreheads, higher than any other animal. Here we collect and assess information from the rest of the brain. We can analyse arguments, imagine the future and plan for it, collaborate with others and several similar behaviours. The frontal lobe can also stop more dangerous and unrealistic behaviours.

Play and creativity also live here, the frontal lobe is connected to the ability to imagine. The fallen tree becomes a pirate ship, or we create something where nothing previously existed - art, reports, a tasty meal.

When we are under stress, this more developed part of the brain will be less active in favour of our more emotional parts. When we are exposed to more noradrenaline in the frontal lobe, the activity in it decreases. This means in practice that we have fewer neurons in the frontal lobe, it can even shrink in size and function less well.

How Graves' Can Affect The Brain

What is behind the impact of the disease on the brain? There are several factors to point out.

T3. Thyroid hormones have a powerful effect on the brain and are found there in relatively high concentrations. T3 regulates important neurotransmitters in the brain, among them serotonin, noradrenaline and adrenaline, and has therefore been linked to depression and anxiety. T3 itself can also act as a neurotransmitter. Most of the T3 found in the brain results from conversion from T4. T4 is transported into the brain and converted in the brain's important support cells, the glial cells, to T3. A smaller proportion, 20 percent, is transported directly in the form of T3.

The brain is sensitive to T3, especially the limbic system that are associate for with your emotions and your wellbeing. No wonder you can feel mentally out of balance with hyperthyroidism. T3 can also create inflammation in the brain and put the nervous system in a stressful situation which is linked to ill health - even mental.

TRH. Acts as a boss over thyroid hormone production and sinks like a rock in Graves'. There is no reason to increase the hormones further, which is why TRH levels go down. Both the brain and the nervous system have to pay for it. TRH increases the activity in the calming part of the nervous system and is a growth factor for the brain and cleanses away oxidation and inflammation. Researchers have linked low TRH to an increased risk of dementia. Treatment with TRH has also been shown to contribute to healing in traumatic brain injuries.

Autoimmunity. Besides the effects of T3, there is the possibility that the symptoms are because of the autoimmune process also affecting the brain. As with ophthalmopathy, TSH receptors in the brain could be targets for the immune system. Antibodies other than TRAb also occur in Graves' and maybe one of them causes an autoimmune attack on the brain.

The nervous system. Lower activity in our calming part of the autonomic nervous system - the parasympathetic nervous system - may be the reason for the negative impact on the limbic system.

Spotlight on: Mental health

Mental illness is linked to thyroid disease. Even when Doctor Robert Graves' first described the disease in the 19th century, great emphasis was placed on mental symptoms. Up to 30 percent of us with Graves' show symptoms of depression at diagnosis. Conversely, many times, unbalanced thyroid hormone levels can also be found in people with depression. Therefore, it is important that the right blood samples are taken when a person seeks care and shows signs of not feeling well mentally. Too often, our mental and physical well-being is divided into two and treated separately when there is mostly an overlap.

Like other diseases associated with Graves', the effect on mental illness remains most times even after hormone levels have returned to normal. The presence of stress has been linked to mental illness remaining, despite stable hormones. Feeling bad mentally can also worsen your Graves'. Therefore, it is important to look at how the mind and the body are connected during treatment.

Mental illnesses are multifactorial, they do not have only one cause. Basically, there are psychosocial factors: difficult life events, trauma, stress in everyday life, relationships and networks, plus our personalities also play a role in triggering and exacerbating mental illness. These factors translate to our individual biochemistry, where also genetics has a role. One of several biological explanatory models that exist - and this is the one treatment with most antidepressant drugs is based on - says that imbalances in the brain's neurotransmitters such as noradrenaline and serotonin contribute to mental illness. The effects of lifestyle change reveal that depression is largely influenced by how we live. For example, proper diet and nutrition, exercise and recovery can prevent or ease depressive symptoms. Mental illness and symptoms associated with Graves':

- Depression
- Anxiety
- Panic attacks
- Bipolar disease
- Thyrotoxic psychosis.

Other diseases affecting the brain associated with Graves':

- Dementia, including Alzheimer's disease.

When the brain is in balance, serotonin and noradrenaline are so too, which stabilizes the mood. When levels fluctuate in the brain, the risk of depression and anxiety increases. T3 can regulate both these neurotransmitters. When serotonin decreases in the brain, the hypothalamus is stimulated to release TRH, which increases TSH and thus the levels of T4 and T3 go up. In depressed patients without thyroid disease, T4 levels in the upper part of the reference range can often be seen. These normalize as depression improves. In hyperthyroidism, serotonin levels are elevated, and normally decrease with treatment.

A study done in Denmark shows that for every 6 months you have had a TSH that is too low, the risk of the most common types of dementia increases by 16 percent. The researchers emphasize the importance of taking action early. One of the most effective things you can do for your brain health is to have a healthy lifestyle. In his book "The End of Alzheimer's", Dale Bredesen has listed 30 causes of dementia and how you can influence them with your lifestyle.

The limbic and nervous system in Graves'

Stress has negative effects on the limbic system. T3 in too high levels can be said to be a stress factor in that the hormone increases the sensitivity to adrenaline. Internal and external stressors can drive the limbic system to create some of the effects we usually see during stress. Do you recognize yourself in any of the following symptoms that the limbic system has been affected by stress?

- Brain fog or inability to concentrate or focus
- Fatigue and low energy
- Chronic muscle and/or joint pain
- Elevated sensory impressions, including smell, taste, light and sound
- Sensitivity to perfumes, detergents or hygiene products
- Anxiety, worry, mood swings or panic attacks
- Depression
- Sleeping problems
- Headache
- Ruminating on past negative events or worries about upcoming events
- Problems with short-term memory or other cognitive problems.

Chronic stress can be seen in the limbic system as the hippocampus becomes less active and even shrinks. The amygdala also changes in size, studies have shown that the size can both increase and decrease. This imbalance causes the symptoms above.

Researching Graves' and the traces it leaves in the brain

Helena Filipsson Nyström, endocrinologist and chief physician at Sahlgrenska University Hospital and associate professor at Sahlgrenska Academy, leads a research group that investigates how the brain is affected in Graves'.

Helena Filipsson Nyström treats patients with Graves' and has with her own seen eyes the mental fatigue the patients describe. The symptoms are similar of those in burnout, according to Helena Filipsson Nyström in an interview with the Swedish Thyroid Association. Patients may also have problems with memory, ability to concentrate and multitasking, anxiety and mood swings. In standard care, there are no elements to rehabilitate the patients' brains, other than general supportive treatment.

Hardly any patients are lucky enough to meet an endocrinologist who knows how Graves' affects the brain. For many doctors, the problem is unknown, and patients receive no information about how the symptoms are related to the disease and how they can be managed. The research group at

Sahlgrenska feel a need to take a closer look at what happens in the brain in Graves'. The goal is to find new treatments.

"At present, I tell my patients with residual problems that it is wise to adapt their life according to their energy levels and what they can do" says Helena Filipsson Nyström to the Thyroid Association.

Helena Filipsson Nyström hopes that with the help of research she will be able to offer a treatment for the problems, but she says that a lot of work remains.

In the so-called CogThy study led by Helena Filipsson Nyström, 65 patients were examined first when they had high hormone levels and then when they were normal. Patients underwent extensive testing with neuropsychological and neuropsychiatric assessments, blood tests and various examinations of the brain. They were also compared with a matching control group.

The Gothenburg group's study could confirm that Graves' patients had more depression, anxiety and mental fatigue than the control group. After 15 months, many still had symptoms. Patients with eye symptoms and a history of mental illness were at greater risk of having symptoms related to the brain.

The measurements of the brain confirmed that both the hippocampus and the amygdala were affected. After 15 months, the amygdala was still affected while the hippocampus had regained a size comparable to that of the control group. When the patients were in the acute stage and had just been diagnosed, there was a connection between TRAb and how much the brain had been affected. The higher the levels of TRAb - the more impact on the brain. A more active disease in the form of high

TRAb also prevented the normalization of not only T3 but also the brain.

The study did not investigate the quality of the limbic system's connections to other parts of the brain in Graves'.

The brain under attack

The results from the first study of the brain in Graves' prompted the Gothenburg group to ask additional questions. About how the immune system and the cognitive symptoms are connected. In an interview in connection with the research receiving a large grant sum, Helena Filipsson Nyström said:

"Our hypothesis is that the cognitive symptoms are because of the immune system not only affecting the thyroid gland but also the brain. We also believe that this effect could be common to what we see in other autoimmune diseases, such as MS and various rheumatic diseases" she says.

The next step in the project is to recruit an additional 310 patients. This time, they will not only look at autoimmune markers linked to the thyroid gland, but also markers linked to other diseases.

"The idea is to see if there is a similar activation of the immune system in different diseases, which also affect the brain" says Helena Filipsson Nyström.

Autoimmunity in the brain affects millions of people worldwide in diseases such as Multiple Sclerosis, Parkinson's and rheumatoid arthritis. An attack on the nervous system can happen against nerves in the body, nerves in the spinal cord or nerve cells in the brain.

Graves' mainly affects the thyroid gland, but the eyes are also affected by the autoimmune reaction. The researchers at Sahlgrenska suspect that the brain may also be a target for the immune system's attacks. TSH - receptors are found in the limbic system, frontal lobe and the parts dedicated to maintaining our internal environment - the hypothalamus and thalamus.

Paul's story: It was nearly impossible to live with my wife

"My wife and I had bought a boat that was a renovation project. It was large, and we had a common dream of sailing a lot with it during the summer. Soon after the purchase, my wife got rushed and tense in the boat project. About what we should do with the boat and when. Sometimes she could be up at night fixing something or ask me to work on it, even though I had been at work all day. It was the same with other things in our lives, a lot of anger and a lot of trouble. When she was diagnosed and began treatment, the only thing she did was sleep. One day she slept six hours besides the hours she slept during the night. I got sympathy from friends, whose partners had experienced burnout. I had to take all the responsibility at home. In retrospect, I wish that I were invited to a visit with the doctor and received information, or at least that someone said that it will get better. A while after she was diagnosed, we understood that the fatigue would be something we had to live with for a while. Now she can do more at home, but a lot is still up to me and our social life is largely put on ice. We got the boat in the water and have sailed with it, even though it was not as renovated as we hoped. I see how she struggles to feel better and I admire her for that, even though it can be difficult to give her a lot of free time every weekend when I would also need it. Graves' is an enormous pressure for the relationship. I can imagine that many couples separate both because of how it is before diagnosis and also after."

*

Graves' kidnaps your personality

The part of the brain that can most closely be described as "yourself" is the frontal lobe. There we find many of the qualities we would like to associate with our personality.

Many with Graves' say that they do not recognize themselves. You are not as good at regulating emotions or control your behaviour. It also becomes more difficult to plan and resolve conflicts.

You do not always have the ability to see how this affects those dear to you. The frontal lobe should normally regulate our impulsivity and help us plan. It has a special task to stand for calm and considered action in various situations.

To test how well the frontal lobe works, you can use dice games for money, The Game of Dice test. Well, not actual money but virtual in a computer game. If you take part, you will be instructed that the goal of the game is to win as much money as possible. On the screen you see two piles of cards, one contains cards with potentially high winnings but also cards where you lose money. The second pile yields low but reliable profits. You do not know the characteristics of the piles in advance but discover them as you play. People with a well-functioning frontal lobe rarely take excessive risks but are content with a reasonable profit by preferring the pile of low, reliable profits. When patients with Graves' took the test, they chose mainly the risky pile during the game, which shows that the function of the frontal lobe is affected.

Autonomic nervous system

When you sweat on a hot summer day or get scared by a thriller movie, the autonomic nervous system is involved. If the limbic system processes our emotions and thoughts, the autonomic nervous system is its messenger. The autonomic nervous system has three important functions:

- Maintain the body's internal environment
- Coordinate the body's response to physical activity and stress
- Help the hormonal system.

Internal organs, such as the heart and lungs, blood vessels and hormone glands are all regulated in whole or in part by the autonomic nervous system. There are three parts of the autonomic nervous system: sympathetic, parasympathetic, and enteric. Sympathetic nervous system is associated with what we usually call "fight or flight", and parasympathetic nervous system stands for "rest and digest".

Sympathetic nervous system. In a stressful situation the sympathetic nervous system is activated. The adrenal glands receive lightning-fast signals to pump out adrenaline, and it prepares your body to escape or fend for your life. The body works hard, and the blood is partially redirected from the internal organs to the muscles. These are more important when the situation is acute. The sympathetic part will take care of the energy reserves and handle crisis situations.

Parasympathetic nervous system. Conversely, if you are in a calm and comfortable situation, you can instead trust that the parasympathetic nervous system is activated. The organs receive signals that the situation is stable, and they can start working with, for example, digestion. When the parasympathetic part is activated, the body is in a state of rest and recovery and the body can get rid of waste products. You feel good when it dominates, you want to play and interact with others.

Enteric nervous system. Nerves around the digestive organs survey the environment there and regulate blood pressure, bowel movements, secretions and fluid transport. It receives both parasympathetic and sympathetic nerve signals.

The vagus nerve

From the brain stem a nerve called the vagus nerve stretches out into the body. Vagus is Latin and means "wanderer", precisely because it is so long that it reaches all the internal organs of the body. It is an especially important part of the parasympathetic nervous system. It is estimated that the vagus nerve accounts for 75 percent of all parasympathetic activity, so you understand what a big role it plays in making us feel relaxed. The vagus nerve collects information from the body and carries it to the brain and sends out information from the brain to the body.

Your brain and intestines work closely together, and the gut can communicate with the brain via the vagus. The intestine is technically part of the outside of the body, and here it can sample its surroundings. The guts' own nervous system, the enteric nervous system is itself large enough to be called "the second brain". When the brain wants to contact the enteric nervous system, it activates the brainstem at the bottom of the brain, which activates the vagus nerve, and finally stimulates the enteric nervous system. The enteric nervous system activates the muscles around the intestines and moves the food forward in the gastrointestinal tract. Therefore, a sign of a weakened vagus nerve may be constipation and overgrowth of unwanted bacteria (which can cause Small Intestinal Bacterial Overgrowth - SIBO) or IBS-like symptoms. 80 percent of the information sent in the vagus goes in the brain's direction. The brain is clearly interested in what the vagus has to say. Vagus is anti-inflammatory, when it is active, the pro-inflammatory signalling in the intestine decreases. When gastrointestinal health is not at its peak, we have unbalanced intestinal flora or leaky gut, the brain perceives it. Inflammatory molecules leak into the blood and reach the brain, and the vagus nerve senses the environment in the intestine and informs the brain about it.

Tone of the autonomic nervous system

Because the vagus is the largest part of our calming nervous system, it will determine if you are in so-called sympathetic or parasympathetic dominance. Both parts of the autonomic nervous system are always activated but the part that is mostly active will dominate. If we look again at the functions of the two parts, we understand why one is healthier for us in the long run than the other.

The sympathetic nervous system, on the one hand, quickly mobilizes your resources for escape or combat, which is detrimental to the body in the long run.

The parasympathetic nervous system is the healing part of the nervous system. Here we heal and rest, a strong vagus helps your body and brain to relax after stress. An active vagus nerve also suppresses inflammation and has been shown to reduce the symptoms of rheumatoid arthritis by reducing the production of inflammatory mediators. There is a positive feedback loop between vagal tone, physical health, and positive emotions. This means that if you support your vagus nerve and improve its function, you will also feel better.

The parts of the autonomic nervous system are usually said to have a tone, a result of how active they are. The tone gives a constant effect on the organs and the body. Which the dominant system is depends, but for the sake of health we should mostly be in parasympathetic dominance. If we have been dominated by the sympathetic nervous system for a long time, it can be measured by a reduction in vagus nerve tone.

We have the image that the heartbeat is always the same, but a healthy nervous system means that the length of the heartbeat varies. It provides a heart rate variability - which is abbreviated HRV. When you measure HRV, you get to know specifically the activity in the part of the vagus that activates the heart, but it is well recognized that this can be generalized to general vagal tone. The heart rate should not vary too much, but not too little either. Decreased tone in the vagus can be measured in the form of HRV going down. HRV is a powerful measure of your health and can estimate your life expectancy. Low HRV can be seen in stress-related illness, cardiovascular disease, depression and many more conditions. HRV is a powerful predictor of future heart health. If you have a vagus nerve in good shape, you will live longer and feel better.

How the autonomic nervous system and the limbic system are connected

Julian Thayer, an expert on the autonomic nervous system and psychologist, has said: "HRV is important not for what it says about the condition of the heart - but about the condition of the brain". The limbic system, the autonomic nervous system, the thyroid gland and your adrenal glands are closely linked to help you overcome and resist stress. The vagus nerve is connected to the brainstem and helps the brain to switch between "fight or flight" and "rest and digest". The brain stem is also connected to the limbic system, so the activity of the autonomic nervous system affects the limbic areas. The brain connects other parts of the limbic system (such as the amygdala and hippocampus) with the autonomic nervous system in two areas of the brain called the insula and cingulum. Here, experiences are translated into action. Widely unique experiences such as nausea, thirst, pain, sexual arousal, anger and heat can all activate this part of the brain. When the signals are weighed together in the insula and cingulum, they become comprehensible, we understand how we should react to what we are experiencing.

Examples of bodily signals to the insula and cingulum can be a calm breathing or a low blood sugar. Thought signals can be anxiety or joy. Environmental signals are, for example, that we see someone we love and are safe with or a tiger who comes running towards us. Insula and cingulum can sense what needs there are the "fight or flight" or it can activate the vagus and we end up in the "rest and digest".

That the insula and cingulum connect body and mind became clear in a study with healthy volunteers. Using brain imaging, the researchers measured the activity of the limbic system, while the subjects could look at photos of emotional faces. It could be happy, scared, or neutral faces. Participants with more anxiety had limbic systems that could not respond as well to the images compared to the controls. It was also found that participants whose brains did not respond to the images also had a lower HRV, that is - a less active vagus nerve.

Graves' and the Vagus Nerve

It is known what happens to the vagus nerve when we get Graves' disease. Studies have been able to measure that HRV is lowered when we are diagnosed. At diagnosis, our vagus nerve is weakened and cannot support our well-being. Blood T3 levels are inversely related to HRV. The higher T3 - the worse HRV. This may be corrected by itself and a better tone of the vagus nerve n measured in most patients after they have returned to normal hormone levels. But does HRV improve in everyone? Do you have symptoms suggestive of reduced HRV perhaps your parasympathetic nervous system has not recovered? Symptoms that your autonomic nervous system is out of balance:

- Irritable Bowel Syndrome (IBS)
- Small Intestinal Bacterial Overgrowth (SIBO)
- Depression
- Anxiety
- Chronic fatigue
- High or low heart rate
- Difficulties swallowing
- Difficulties falling asleep in the evening or waking up at night
- Gastroparesis, the gut does not empty
- Heartburn and acid reflux
- Dizziness/fainting
- B12 deficiency
- Chronic inflammation
- Weight problems.

The effects of T3 to promote the sympathetic nervous system is an important reason HRV is lowered in Graves'. The absence of TRH also plays a role because it can activate the vagus nerve in the brainstem. When researchers studied the effects of TRH on experimental animals, they saw that several of the functions we associate with vagus, such as secreting gastric acid and bowel movements, increase when the animals receive TRH. When we do not have hyperthyroidism, this is a marvellous example of the balance the body always strives for. When T3 further down the physiological chain promotes the sympathetic part of the autonomic nervous system, TRH higher up has already activated the vagus which works as a counterweight. But for us with Graves', it becomes a double blow to our healing and soothing parasympathetic nervous system when hormone levels are raised without the feedback loop working. TRH drops which leads to the vagus not being stimulated and because T3 is constantly high, it spurs on the sympathetic nervous system.

CHAPTER 6

TIRED ADRENALS

Freya's story: Resting did not help my fatigue

"When I had just gotten my diagnosis, I mostly just wanted to get the drugs so I could continue my life as usual. My plan was to take the four weeks of sick leave I was offered and then get back to full time at work. I can tell you this: It did not go as planned. After four weeks, I had not even found my dose of the drugs and had just realized how sick I was. Sick leave was extended for a while. Above all, I was so tired. I just wanted to sleep, but I did not make me any more alert or energized. Despite that, I did not let go of my idea of rushing back to work. I felt like a traitor when I was home and on sick leave. In retrospect, I wish I had taken my time and asked for more sick leave because I needed it."

*

The adrenal glands distribute the energy during the day

Together with the thyroid gland, the adrenal glands help us meet the body's need for energy. Some resemble the thyroid gland with a car's accelerator and the adrenal glands with the gearbox. Both are needed to determine the speed at which the car moves forward. We find the adrenal glands as small caps on top of the kidneys and they are important hormone glands. They produce several hormones, including cortisol and noradrenaline. That the adrenal gland and the thyroid gland are connected can also be seen in the circadian rhythm of the respective hormones. At night, T3 is at its lowest and then peaks before it is time for us to wake up. The T3 peak causes the adrenal glands to secrete cortisol which helps us to wake up and feel energized in the morning. When the adrenal glands cannot produce enough hormone for our needs or the circadian rhythm is disrupted, they cannot support our health as they should.

What is stress?

The word stress may make you think of having a lot to do, an impossible schedule where you are just not able to do it all. But more things can strain the body, and especially the adrenal glands. Different types of stress:

- Cold or hot temperatures
- Internal stress from low self-esteem or anxiety
- Diseases such as infections, autoimmune disease or other chronic diseases
- Trauma or emergencies
- Pain
- Fluctuating blood sugar or too low energy intake
- Caffeine and nicotine are stimulants and releases stress hormones, some are also sensitive to chocolate and tea containing the same family of compounds
- Too much to do, even if it is fun activities.

Cortisol-not (only) a bad guy

Cortisol has gained a reputation for being a "bad" hormone because, among other effects, high levels can increase the storage of belly fat and affect the brain negatively. Actually, it is an amazing survival mechanism the body has. Without cortisol, we could not balance vital functions such as blood sugar, blood pressure, or the immune system. It may just as well be called a survival hormone. Cortisol interacts with both thyroid hormones and sex hormones. Adequate levels of cortisol can make you feel happy waking up in the morning, focused and full of energy. Cortisol is something normal and necessary and only becomes bad for us when we are exposed to high levels for a long time. In Graves', T3 is unnaturally high, which can cause the adrenal glands to burn out by forming and releasing cortisol at a furious rate. By supporting the adrenal glands, you can facilitate their recovery.

The HPA axis

When the brain perceives something that is stressing it, signals are sent to the hypothalamus in the brain to release a hormone called corticotropin-releasing hormone (CRH). Stress should be perceived in the broadest sense of the word and can include everything from inflammatory mediators from the immune system to a crazy boss with unreasonable demands. CRH signals to the pituitary gland to produce the hormone ACTH, which it then sends out into the bloodstream. Cortisol is formed and released in the adrenal cortex when ACTH reaches the adrenal glands. The time until we see elevated cortisol levels in the blood after stress is about 15 minutes and the levels can stay elevated for several hours. These three hormonal glands together: the hypothalamus, the pituitary gland, and the adrenal glands are also called the HPA axis. Adrenaline and noradrenaline are formed and released instantaneously into the bloodstream through the immediate activation of the sympathetic nervous system by stress. Then adrenaline can have its effects as a hormone. When cortisol rises in the blood, the brain "reads" it and should then stop producing CRH, as a signal to the body not to produce more cortisol. A constant high level of cortisol in the blood is not normal and the brain then has this natural feedback system that should turn off the impulses to produce more.

The HPA axis in Graves'

Cortisol and the adrenal glands are often affected in Graves'. Usually, the thyroid gland and the adrenal glands communicate with each other, and when the levels of cortisol become too high, it can suppress the thyroid hormones. The thyroid hormones can increase adrenal activity in the form of increased production in the adrenal medulla and turnover of cortisol in the liver.

T3 can increase ACTH in the brain which stimulates the adrenal gland, and T3 can increase the production of the enzymes that break down cortisol in the liver. In Graves', communication and feedback loops are put out of play, the brain does not receive the signal to reduce cortisol. The thyroid gland keeps pumping out hormones, which causes the adrenal glands to work hard.

Not only do the adrenal glands release cortisol on more occasions during the day than normal, a larger part of the day the adrenal gland is also in a secretory phase, more cortisol is produced, and more is also broken down.

A common test to check the function of the adrenal glands is to inject a dose of the hormone that stimulates them, ACTH. Blood samples are then taken to measure the amount of cortisol released from the adrenal gland. Once you have had Graves' for a while, the secretion can be significantly lower, especially at diagnosis. The adrenal glands have lost their reserves and cannot do their normal functions. Approximately 10 percent of all Graves' patients have adrenal insufficiency at diagnosis - the secretion of cortisol is less than the body's needs.

Do you have symptoms related to the adrenal glands?

Symptoms when the adrenal glands are not working properly can be many. First, we have a group of symptoms in the phase when the adrenal glands are working at full capacity, then the stage enters when they lose their capacity. Finally, we end up in the situation when they cannot produce enough cortisol.

Wired. When the adrenal glands work more than normal, you may experience a stage where you feel "wired". If you can quickly identify that the symptoms are coming from the adrenal glands, you prevent slipping into the other stages:

- Eating large amounts of food in the evening
- Weight gain that sticks on the belly
- The feeling of running in a hamster wheel all day
- High anxiety or panic attacks
- Feelings of anger, depression, or frustration
- Difficulties to fall asleep or wake up at night

- Difficulties to focus and concentrate
- PMS or problems with menstruation, perimenopause, or menopause
- Low sex drive.

Wired and tired. In the second phase, you recognize several of the symptoms from the "wired" phase. It can be confusing that you now see symptoms that almost contradict your previous symptoms, the phase is therefore called "wired and tired". This is because the adrenal glands are now decreasing their production of hormone or the circadian rhythm of the secretion is disturbed. Common symptoms in this phase:

- Addicted to caffeine to get through the day
- Hard to wake up in the morning
- Tired during the day
- Low sex drive
- Weight gain
- Waking up with high anxiety
- Digestive problems
- Frustration, anger or depression
- Hard to fall asleep
- Hair loss
- Weakened immune system
- Dizziness or low blood pressure
- Craving for salt.

Tired. If you ignore the previous phases, you may end up in the last stage of adrenal imbalance - "tired". Symptoms of this phase include:

- Complete loss of energy
- Unexplained weight gain you cannot get rid of, whatever you do
- Addicted to caffeine to function somewhat
- Blood sugar imbalances
- Extreme craving for salty or sweet foods, or refined carbs
- Feeling tired even after sleeping all night
- Low sex drive

- The slightest challenge feels overwhelming, you react badly to stress
- Mild depression
- Brain fog.

Spotlight on: Chronic infections

From the chapter on calming the immune system, you remember that infections with certain bacteria and viruses, especially coxsackie virus, Yersinia enterocolitica, Borrelia burgdorferi, Helicobacter pylori and retroviruses (HTLV-1, HFV, HIV and SV40) and hepatitis C can trigger Graves'. Viruses or bacteria create imbalances in the immune system, which increases the risk of autoimmunity. The immune reaction also creates inflammation, which is also a risk factor. Finally, we have "molecular mimicry", some bacteria and viruses are similar to proteins in the thyroid gland, so their presence triggers a reaction against your own body. When the immune system cannot cure an infection, it becomes chronic. Viruses or bacteria remain more or less active in the body. In the list above with viruses and bacteria often found in Graves', we have several that are known for becoming chronic. Chronic infections can maintain the autoimmune reaction by the virus or bacterium resembling your own tissue. This leads the immune system to attack itself. An infection also causes the immune system to secrete pro-inflammatory mediators that circulate throughout the body and lay the foundation of autoimmune disease. Inflammation is a stress to the body, which places higher demands on the adrenal glands. When the adrenal glands' reserves and function are reduced, the immune system is affected by cortisol taking a step back from its regulatory role. An altered circadian rhythm in cortisol secretion has also been linked to increased activity of autoimmune diseases. If you suspect a chronic infection, seek help from a skilled practitioner. Also use lifestyle measures in this book that are immune-boosting and therefore help to cure infections: nutritious diet, less stress, more sleep and increased physical activity.

Affected circadian rhythm impairs sleep

Sleeping well is crucial for mental and physical health. We need about 7 to 8 hours of sleep per night for health and to feel well. Ill health - even mental - is very much linked to the effect of a disrupted circadian rhythm. This connection probably goes both ways, that is - you can sleep poorly because you have mental illness, but you can also suffer from mental illness because you sleep poorly. For example, sleep problems increase the risk of depression. Poor sleep is also a risk factor for cardiovascular disease and other common diseases.

Getting good sleep can be complicated when you have adrenals and thyroid glands that are not working properly. Cortisol controls the circadian rhythm and is at its lowest at night before it rises in the morning. Without this marking of the circadian rhythm, sleep can deteriorate and we need a lot of sleep to help the body and the adrenal glands recover.

Sleep and limbic system are closely related. Sleep problems are associated with an overactive limbic system, both during wakefulness and during the sleep period. Differences in brains in people with good and poor sleep can be seen in brain imaging. Sleeping is also one of the most anti-inflammatory things we can do. Disturbed night's sleep has been linked to an increased risk of autoimmune diseases. It has been shown that when people with poor sleep improve it, the risk of autoimmune disease decreases.

The adrenal glands miss their building block cholesterol

Cholesterol has an undeserved bad reputation. The bad reputation is due to the fact that it appears at high levels at the same time as inflammatory conditions - but it is not the cause of disease. In cardiovascular disease, cholesterol levels have been linked to an increased risk of, for example, a heart attack. But if you look behind the curtain of this connection, you see that cardiovascular disease is not caused by cholesterol. Or as the researchers behind a study on cholesterol and inflammation put it: "Inflammation, not cholesterol, causes chronic disease". Cholesterol is instead something positive and necessary for us to have adequate levels of.

We use it to build cell membranes, heal injuries, create hormones like estrogen, testosterone and cortisol, as an antioxidant and precursor to Vitamin D. We get cholesterol in our diet but can also form it ourselves. When we eat cholesterol, the body forms less of its own. Misunderstandings about cholesterol arose in the last century when researchers assumed that high cholesterol caused cardiovascular disease. These ideas are being questioned more and more. As an example, the Framingham Heart study, a study on risk factors for cardiovascular disease, could not link cholesterol intake to a higher risk of cardiovascular disease. Other studies have shown that older people with high cholesterol live longer. Studies have also shown that treatment that only reduces inflammation, without lowering cholesterol - reduces the risk of cardiovascular disease.

Low cholesterol may instead be harmful. A Danish study could see that individuals with low levels of cholesterol had an increased risk of autoimmunity. The researchers behind the Framingham Heart Study have examined data that compared patients' cholesterol levels with their cognitive abilities. Almost 2000 people, women and men, underwent tests that showed how well their memory, learning ability, conceptualization, concentration, attention, organizational skills and abstract thinking worked every four to six years. In 2005, researchers reported that lower cholesterol levels were linked to impaired cognitive abilities. This is in line with other studies that show that low cholesterol levels are linked to depression and dementia. Cholesterol is an important nutrient for the brain, even essential for its function. The brain needs cholesterol in large amounts but cannot produce it itself in any sizeable amount. It must therefore be transported into the brain.

What then happens to cholesterol in Graves'? More cholesterol is produced in the liver, but more is also used and overall, the levels decrease, which can affect inflammation, hormone balance and brain health negatively. When TSH rises again, cholesterol can get back to normal levels. Cholesterol is normalized in most patients with Graves' two months after normal thyroid hormone levels are reached.

Eye disease and cholesterol

For patients with eye disease, the story is different, often you have elevated levels of the cholesterol that is usually seen in other inflammatory conditions. Graves' eye disease probably means a more activated immune system, which leads to increased inflammation and oxidative stress in the eye. Something that leads to fluid accumulation and growth of tissue in the eye socket. Researchers believe that the elevated cholesterol level in Graves' eye disease may be caused by an underlying inflammatory condition.

The most common drug for lowering cholesterol are statins. Many claim that treatment with statins does not address the actual problem (which is inflammation) and has side effects, including damaging our mitochondria and weakening the immune system. The statins reduce the body's own production of cholesterol. However, it has been seen that treatment with statins can be a protection against developing eye disease in Graves'. This is probably because statins do more than lower cholesterol. It can inhibit the formation of fat cells and cells that produce supporting tissue in the eye and act as an antioxidant. There is no study that has investigated whether an anti-inflammatory lifestyle could affect the risk of getting eye disease or reducing symptoms you already have. A diet with an anti-inflammatory effect has reduced the risk of diseases where elevated cholesterol levels are usually seen. From the chapter on inflammation, you also remember that symptoms of eye disease can be reduced by antioxidants. The conclusion is that it is not cholesterol you should worry about in eye disease, but find ways to reduce autoimmunity and inflammation.

Adrenal glands on overdrive steal hormone building blocks

Cortisol and our sex hormones, testosterone, estrogen and progesterone come from the same building block: cholesterol. From cholesterol, pregnenolone is formed and from there we can form the other hormones. Environmental factors can affect whether pregnenolone should become cortisol or any of the other hormones. Maybe you can guess which environmental factor can determine the faith of pregnenolone? Stress. When we experience stress, the body will form less of the anabolic, healing hormones such as testosterone or estrogen and instead form cortisol. This is often called "pregnenolone steal" and means that the precursor to our long-term beneficial hormones is stolen by the body's acute stress response.

The result can be that we get different symptoms because of low levels of sex hormones. The brain also does not get the amount of beneficial hormones it needs, which can aggravate the problems Graves' has already caused. The sex hormones are vital for the brain and lower levels have been linked to altered levels of neurotransmitters, depression, difficulty sleeping and dementia. Fluctuations in hormones have been associated with a lower quality of life at menopause.

One way to find out if pregnenolone is going to produce cortisol or sex hormones is to measure the levels of the hormone dehydroepiandrosterone in is sulphated version (DHEA-S) in the blood. DHEA-S has beneficial actions on its own and is a precursor to other hormones. It is formed in the adrenal glands and converted in the testes or ovaries to testosterone and estrogen. DHEA-S is sometimes described as a miracle cure for counteracting aging, as its production decreases steadily from the age of 20. That is probably to promise too much, but the hormone has many beneficial effects to keep the body and brain healthy. There is a positive correlation between levels of DHEA-S and good cognition in both men and women, highlighting its role in strengthening our limbic system.

The levels of DHEA-S are reduced in Graves', which confirms that we risk losing not only the beneficial effects of DHEA-S but also our sex hormones. Examples of symptoms of hormonal imbalances in men of all ages:

- Low sex drive
- Fluctuations in brain function, focus and mood
- Lost muscle mass
- Sweating.

Examples of symptoms of hormonal imbalances in women before menopause:

- Menstrual cycle length varies
- Hot flashes and sweating attacks
- Low sex drive
- Sleeping problems
- Fluctuations in brain function, focus and mood.

Examples of symptoms of hormonal imbalances in menopausal women:

- Dryness and discomfort in the vagina, urinary tract infections
- Hot flashes and sweating attacks
- Low sex drive
- Sleeping problems
- Fluctuations in brain function, focus and mood.

Why am I always tired? I feel more like I have hypothyroidism.

More thyroid hormone should give more energy, one might think. And maybe that is true during the initial stages of the disease. But as time goes on, the body is affected by constantly going at full speed. Nutrients are running out, the mitochondria's rapid energy production is leaking inflammatory mediators, adrenal glands that cannot produce cortisol, and constant poor sleep also drain us of energy. And with the alarm button jammed in the nervous system, that means that we never really get to calm down, which makes us more tired. The net effect is reduced energy.

Am I burned out?

Many of us with Graves' have asked ourselves if we are suffering from burnout. Stress resistance is low and fatigue is paralyzing. Sometimes the disease pushes us over the edge, and we get burnout. If you do, you should be treated for it.

CHAPTER 7
MUSCLE AND BONE ARE BROKEN DOWN

Muscle strength, the amount of muscle mass you have and the number of minutes you exercise are all linked to a higher quality of life. We humans are built for movement, getting where we want to go by walking or running. We also feel good when we move our bodies.

When your muscles get bigger and bones get stronger, you are in anabolic phase. The opposite is when tissues instead breaks down. Maybe we do not use our muscles and bones in a stimulating way, that we get older or are stressed. Stress causes the body to break down tissue to take the stored energy and nutrients to use during more urgent needs. What is the point of maintaining your strength if you die today, the body seems to reason.

It is not the size of the muscles that is most important for a positive impact on health. Rather, it is the strength of your muscles that helps you stay healthy.

Movement and resistance are a signal for muscles and bones to get stronger. For this to happen, the tissues need the right building blocks in the form of nutrients. The nutrition is also needed for us to exercise. Muscle weakness can affect a muscle or the entire body. If you experience symptoms of muscle weakness, it is best to reverse it with exercise. If you need to, you can seek the help of a physiotherapist. Here are some symptoms of weakened muscles:

- Difficulties to perform daily tasks such as opening jars or carrying grocery bags
- Problems with balance

- Fatigue and lack of energy
- Cannot lift as heavy things as before
- Trying to train but it is too hard.

Graves' can affect muscles

When you have high thyroid levels, your metabolism increases to sky-high levels, which becomes debilitating to you. This has consequences for the parts of the body that relate to movement: heart, muscles and skeleton.

For example, the function of the heart can change and you risk beating it too fast, raising blood pressure and even heart failure. With Graves', the heart gets an increased sensitivity to the stress hormone noradrenaline, which leads to it working very hard. The heart is an important reason that in the beginning after diagnosis you should be careful with exercise as it also strains the heart. You will learn later on in the chapter on exercise how to know when you are ready for it.

The muscles account for 30 to 40 percent of the resting metabolism, so the increased energy consumption in Graves' is mostly because of the increased turnover of energy in the muscles. The increased metabolism leads to them showing signs of increased breakdown, and this breakdown is directly linked to the status of the thyroid gland. This causes a loss of muscle mass and muscle strength. Besides weakness, several other symptoms from the musculoskeletal system associated with Graves' can appear: frozen shoulder, Dupuytren's contracture, trigger finger, decreased joint mobility and carpal tunnel syndrome. It is therefore important to know that Graves' can be a contributing cause of any symptoms from joints and muscles and seek physical therapy. In drug treatment, weight loss is reversed and the initial weight gain is mostly muscle. One study tested the strength of the muscles and found that it was reduced at diagnosis but returned during drug treatment with beta-blockers and was back to normal levels after 6 months when the patients' thyroid hormones were normal again. There is a natural recovery for most of us here too, the body is fantastic at healing itself.

The skeleton is also affected in Graves'

The skeleton is in a constant process of building and breakdown. This is normal, and the important thing is the net effect on the bone mass. Is breakdown or building factors predominant? In Graves', the turnover of bone mass increases and the bone is broken down, which can also be seen by calcium excreted in higher levels than usual with the urine. The bone mass decreases and the risk of fractures increases and remains high even 5 years after the hyperthyroidism, especially for woman who have gone through menopause. The skeleton of women before menopause is also influenced. A Danish study that followed women with Graves' before menopause and their bone density could show that at diagnosis, bone density was reduced. Also, compared to patients who had Hashimoto's. Bone density then increased during drug treatment. TRAb and free T4, that is how active the disease was, could predict how large the loss of bone mass was. Thereafter, the researchers could see that after drug treatment, up to 18 months after, bone density decreased again. The researchers could not say what the reduction after treatment was caused by, perhaps that some women got higher thyroid hormone levels again.

For men, it is not yet clear what effect Graves' has on bone mass. TSH sinks in Graves' and normally it protects the skeleton by stimulating bone formation and preventing degradation. Stress hormones and inflammation are negative for bone. Early treatment with beta-blockers can limit the amount of bone mass lost.

If you have other risk factors for bone thinning, besides Graves', really make sure to counteract the loss of bones with lowering inflammation in combination with the right exercise and nutrition. Other risk factors for bone thinning:

- Old age, menopause for women
- Some types of previous fractures
- Heredity
- BMI <20 or weight loss> 22 lbs or 10 kg since the age of 25
- Tall stature
- Smoking
- Rheumatoid arthritis
- Physical inactivity
- Stumbles often, problems with balance
- Cortisone treatment
- Treatment with hypnotics, benzodiazepines and SSRIs.

Spotlight on: Osteoporosis

Bone thinning is also called osteoporosis and is a potentially fatal disease. You can get bone fractures more easily if you have osteoporosis and weaker bones. The most common are bone fractures in the wrists, hips, spine or upper arms. Osteoporosis is due to the fact that the balance between the breakdown and building up of bones in the body is disturbed, so that more bone mass is broken down than is regenerated. Behind osteoporosis is often an inflammation that erodes the skeleton, which is why it is linked to many other common diseases. Osteoporosis is most common in postmenopausal women. This is because of the reduced sex hormone estrogen which is a powerful protective factor for the skeleton. But becoming osteoporotic has begun long before that. Up to the age of 30, we build bone mass and then it breaks down faster than it builds up. Throughout our lives, we need to make sure that the skeleton is kept strong. You will learn more about how this is done in part three of the book.

The trauma of breaking a bone - especially the hip and subsequent surgery in combination with underlying health problems can increase the risk of dying. Increased risk of dying from hip fractures can also be because of complications after the fracture, such as infections, internal bleeding, stroke or heart failure. Your bone health is other words well worth taking care of.

PART THREE - YOUR ROADMAP TO HEALING

In this section, you will receive suggestions for specific lifestyle changes with the potential to increase your quality of life and help you recover from Graves'. When we feel anxious, tired, stressed and low, often there is not much information offered on what we can do ourselves. But you have enormous power and possibility in using lifestyle to feel better. Starting now.

CHAPTER 8

NEWLY DIAGNOSED? READ THIS FIRST

This book contains many ideas on how you can feel better in Graves'. When you just had your diagnosis, you are probably tired, and your mind is foggy. Then you need some short and concise advice. It all may seem overwhelming and you are in a phase of the disease where your best bet is resting. Try one thing at a time, most important of all is to rest and that you learn to sleep again. This chapter also applies to anyone with Graves' who still feel deeply affected by the disease, with many symptoms of an active stress response. Here is what you need to do now:

Rest. The most important thing right now is to rest as much as you can. Nervous system, brain and adrenal glands have been working at high speed with elevated thyroid hormone levels. Extend your sick leave as long as you have the opportunity to, and talk to family and friends that you now need to recover. Also skip stimulants such as coffee and alcohol on pause. Listen to your body what it wants and what it does not want.

Learn to sleep again. Restoring sleep is important because it enables all other recovery after the illness. Read the chapter on restoring the adrenal glands for practical steps on how to do it.

Reduce stress and anxiety. Save all the big questions about the disease and life for when you are in better balance. Try to reduce anxiety and stress. Give yourself positive impressions, focus on calming and happy thoughts. It will get better, some will have persistent symptoms or eye problems but it does not have to apply to you.

Active recovery for brain and nervous system. You can try breathing exercises and meditation and see if it is rewarding to you. If it does not work at all, you can try again a little later, as these are important tools for the brain and nervous system to be balanced again.

Supply nutrition. Nutrition is drained by the disease so eat nutritious and well, take a high-quality multivitamin supplement (ask a health food store you trust if you are unsure of what to choose). Supplementation with carnitine can block thyroid hormones from entering the cell and supplementation in patients newly diagnosed with Graves' reduces mental and physical fatigue. After beginning treatment, most people gain weight and most of it is muscle mass. There are many who try autoimmune diet protocols, but if it is alien to how you normally eat, it can be a stress for the body to adjust. Go ease, you know your body best.

Antioxidants. A trick you can try for faster recovery is to take supplements with antioxidants such as vitamin E, beta carotene, CoQ10, vitamin C, selenium, glutathione and the minerals copper, zinc and magnesium important for forming the body's own antioxidants. Studies suggest taking antioxidants for two months early after diagnosis, speeds up recovery. Some of the symptoms in Graves' are because high metabolism produces substances that consume antioxidants. Refilling on these can therefore be good, but settle for eight weeks because supplements in the long run prevent the body's own antioxidants from forming. Selenium and Q10 can be continued for a longer period if you wish.

Learn about the disease and your body. Read about the disease and become sensitive to your body. It sends you signals about what it needs. If you have not listened before or heard but still kept going, you need to break that pattern. Your body has not done this to you out of spite, it has happened become ill and now needs your care. You have an excellent opportunity to become an expert on your own body and health.

When you have made some recovery, individually when that happens

After a while, you will hopefully be stable in your thyroid hormones, even if that does not mean that you feel good. If you are not yet stable, your priority is to become so with the help of your doctor. In the meantime, you can take inspiration from the advice above for newly diagnosed patients.

Once you have received your doctor's approval to exercise, do so, given all the health benefits of physical activity. Start slowly and notice how it feels in your body. In the exercise chapter, you get tools to determine what your body is ready for. If you notice that exercise is not yet right for you, you can lean towards sleep, rest, recovery for the brain and nervous system and a nutritious diet to recover further before you increase your exercise. The keywords here are again: Listen to your body.

Lab tests in Graves'

The most important thing when we are not feeling well or tired is to focus on the lifestyle changes above. When, despite a healthy lifestyle, we still do not feel well, there may be a need to do a health test that shows where the imbalances linger. This can be a test of organic acids in the urine, intestinal flora, methylation, inflammation, heart rate variability or nutritional status. You can read more about tests in Appendix A of this book.

CHAPTER 9

SELF ASSESSMENT: CREATE YOUR ROADMAP TO HEALING

You are now ready to create your personal, unique roadmap to healing from Graves' disease. In this chapter are questionnaires for you to use when uncovering what you should focus on facilitating your self-healing. Remember that there is no other healing than self-healing. Your body has an amazing ability to regenerate and restore its health and function. All it asks of you is to provide an environment that allows it to do so.

That is exactly what we are creating here. By answering questions on your lifestyle and symptoms, you will learn how to provide your body with what it needs to activate this function called self-healing. Do not underestimate it.

It is never too late to turn on this superpower, either. Anyone can do something for their health. Some can do more, others less, but the good news is that everything counts. These lifestyle changes will also lower the risk for any other disease. If this road map assessment says you need to move more to reduce symptoms of Graves' then that is what you need to do to decrease risk of type 2 diabetes, heart disease, cancer and mental illness. You get it all in one package.

If you are already edgy about what this book will say you have to do, relax. Later in this chapter, you will learn the ins and outs of how to make new habits. Stick around, because the methods may not be what you think. But first, we will get you assessed. It is time to take a big step towards healing from Graves'.

How to use the questionnaires

These questions show you what lifestyle changes you should focus on to heal from Graves'. For some of us, it is balancing brain and nervous system and for others restoring the adrenal glands is key. It can be all of them.

Read the statements at your own pace. When you find one you resonate with, circle it and at the end - add up all the circles of that grouping. Do not skip any of them, even those who do not seem relevant to you. Some symptoms will be repeated in more than one part, that is a result of the body being a whole - not separate systems working isolated from each other. Finally, what parts that are most important to you will be clear. After the assessments, you will get an explanation of what your results mean.

Do you need to calm your immune system?

1.	I am smoker
2.	I have had infections from EVB, Lyme, Hepatitis C, Coxsackie virus, Borrelia burgdorferi (Lyme disease), H. Pylori or retrovirus (HTLV-1, HFV, HIV and SV40).
3.	I eat algae several times a week, take a supplement with iodine or eat plenty of seafood daily.
4.	I am sedentary, meaning I move less than 30 minutes per day at a pace that makes me sweat.
5.	I have aches and pains that only seem to get worse.
6.	I have one active autoimmune disease or more.

7.	I avoid being in the sunlight or live where it is dark for some time of the year. I do not take D-vitamin supplements or eat fatty fish either.
8.	I am pregnant, have just been pregnant or in menopause.
9.	I have had a negative life event happen to me, such as the death of a loved one, an accident or divorce or live under stressful conditions.
10.	My grip is getting weaker or I am losing muscle.
11.	I regularly take anti-inflammatory medications.
12.	I sleep less than 7 to 8 hours per night or I do not wake up rested in the morning.
13.	I get sick easily and catch everything around.
14.	I get less than 200 mcg of selenium per day.
15.	I am exposed to endocrine disruptors from using a lot of plastics, make up or hygiene products with unknown ingredients, amalgam fillings or flame retardants in furniture or fabrics.
16.	I supplement with melatonin.

0 or below 3 items circled: Awesome, this area is probably not something you need to worry about. Maybe your Graves' disease is in remission or you have a healthy lifestyle. You will still benefit from checking in with the chapter on getting a calm immune system to make sure that this will not become a troublesome area for you.

3 items or above circled: Most likely, your immune system is in some imbalance. It can be scary to think about that you are living a lifestyle that promotes immune dysfunction. But do not get immobilized with fear, instead turn it to your advantage and see all the things you can do to bring balance to the force. Several lifestyle factors are associated

with healing from Graves' or avoiding a relapse. You will learn about them in the chapter on how to calm the immune system.

Do you need to fill up on nutrients?

1.	I eat processed food daily or several times weekly.
2.	I experience stress in my daily life.
3.	I eat fewer than 500 grams fruits and vegetables per day.
4.	My diet comprises several servings of grains each day.
5.	I am a vegetarian or vegan.
6.	My skin and hair look dull.
7.	My energy levels are low.
8.	On my skin there are unexplained rashes.
9.	I eat the same foods every day.
10.	I do not believe taking supplements is necessary.
11.	I do not eat fatty fish or take fish oil supplements.
12.	I drink more than one alcoholic beverage per day.
13.	Sugary foods are a staple for me.
14.	I never use herbs in my cooking.
15.	Cacao or berries are not part of my diet.

0 or below 3 items circled: Awesome, this area is probably not something you need to worry about. You eat enough nutrients to cover your needs. Just to be sure, take a peek at the chapter on nutrition anyway to see if there are any additional ways you can get dialled in.

3 items or above circled: As for so many others, your diet is probably not supporting your health at the moment. Every day, your body uses a lot of different nutrients and many of them we have to get from our diet. Otherwise we risk facing a plethora of symptoms and diseases. But do not fear, this is the most delicious lifestyle intervention and the chapter on nutrition will give you points in the right direction.

Do you need to balance brain or nervous system?

1.	I have an inner feeling of constant stress.
2.	I find it difficult to calm down.
3.	My sleep is shorter than 7 hours per night, disturbed, or I wake up feeling tired.
4.	I spend a lot of time online and with my smartphone.
5.	I never do yoga or meditate.
6.	I do not spend as much time with family members or friends as I wish.
7.	I have depression, anxiety or other mental illness.
8.	My mood is often low or I am anxious about the future.
9.	My internal dialogue is negative.
10.	I find it difficult to find things to be thankful for.
11.	I can hardly remember when was the last time I laughed.
12.	I use cigarettes, alcohol or other substances to wind down.
13.	I have problems with my digestion or IBS.
14.	I eat less than 500 grams of vegetables, berries or herbs per day.
15.	When I think about the future, it feels hopeless.

16.	I have measured my Heart Rate Variability, and it was low.

0 or below 3 items circled: Awesome, this area is probably not something you need to worry about. You are calm, centred and serene-at least most of the time. No doubt you have developed strategies and techniques for achieving this. For some inspiration on other techniques to try in staying relaxed, read the chapter on balancing brain and nervous system.

3 items or above circled: If you are troubled by stress, you are not alone. So many of us have too many things to do and too little time to do them in. That is not even accounting for the things we want to do (like have some unplanned time for ourselves to do whatever we feel like), those we just ignore. Taking time for yourself or mind-body techniques is not an option in today's world - it is a necessity. Therefore, head on over to the chapter on balancing brain and nervous system and choose from the many practices that will help you centre yourself.

Do you need to restore your adrenal glands?

1.	I have disturbed sleep or sleep less than 7 hours per night.
2.	I am always fatigued or feel burnt out.
3.	My cups of coffee get me through the day.
4.	I have big dips of energy in the afternoon.
5.	I have a hard time waking up in the morning.
6.	My life and schedule is busy and I feel pressure from it.
7.	I have depression, anxiety, or other mental illness.
8.	I have had infections or have a chronic infection.

9.	My bones are brittle and I have been told I have, or am at risk for - osteoporosis.
10.	My blood sugar is unstable and I need a sugary snack between or after most meals.
11.	I crave salt or salty foods.
12.	Do you often have colds or flus?
13.	Do you sometimes get dizzy when standing up?
14.	I avoid fat in my diet.
15.	I never eat citrus fruit, kiwi, cruciferous vegetables, or berries.

0 or below 3 items circled: Awesome, this area is probably not something you need to worry about. Your adrenals have restored after the acute phase of the disease and you enjoy stable energy levels throughout your day. If you want to know more about how to give your adrenals, the attention they deserve, look in the chapter on restoring adrenal glands.

3 items or above circled: In Graves' we often have affected adrenals and if we keep stressing them out, they are likely to stay that way. You probably know perfectly well what situations in your life stress you out. If you cannot change them now, besides working on restoring adrenals you can also turn to the chapter on acceptance. Sometimes we need a reminder that how we view the world have a great impact on our energy levels. The chapter on adrenal health also lets you their favourite nutrients, the importance of stabilising blood sugar and more.

Do you need to strengthen muscle and bone?

1.	I do not exercise for 30 minutes per day at a pace that makes me sweat.
2.	I am always fatigued or lack energy.
3.	My protein intake is below 1,8 oz or 50 grams per day.
4.	I have lost muscle mass.
5.	My grip is weaker.
6.	I do not incorporate strength training in my exercise regime.
7.	I do not do brisk walking, running, biking, or another form of cardiovascular exercise.
8.	I never walk or bike to where I am going.
9.	I have had fractures in the past.
10.	I have gone through menopause.
11.	One or more of relatives have had osteoporosis, brittle bones or fracture of arm, hip or foot.
12.	I avoid being in the sunlight or live where it is quite for some time of the year. I do not take D-vitamin supplements or eat fatty fish either.
13.	I am a vegetarian or a vegan.
14.	I do not eat 500 grams of fruits or vegetables per day.
15.	I have aches and pains that only seem to multiply and get worse.

0 or below 3 items circled: Awesome, this area is probably not something you need to worry about. You are strong and can enjoy your body's vitality during your daily tasks. If you want to know more about how get even stronger, look in the chapter on muscle and bone health.

3 items or above circled: Congratulations! You have the possibility of unlocking one of the most powerful lifestyle factors in feeling good – exercise. Maybe you have never exercised or just gotten off track. It does not matter. In the chapter on strengthening muscle and bone you will learn what you need to get into it.

Do you need to adopt an accepting frame of mind?

1.	I think about why this had to happen to me.
2.	I find it hard to find something to be grateful for.
3.	It is impossible for me to accept my situation.
4.	A smile almost never comes across my face.
5.	My internal dialogue is harsh.
6.	I do not even know what the term "listen to your body" really means.
7.	Accepting my situation would be giving up on improving it.
8.	I never question my thoughts as untrue or unrealistic.
9.	I assume others are much freer of suffering than me.
10.	I never share my thoughts or feelings on experiencing these symptoms.
11.	I cannot say I like myself and believe in it.
12.	Compassion is not something I value or practice.
13.	Anyone who will accept being ill is weak.
14.	If I am not free of these symptoms soon, all my efforts will be worthless.

15.	If I do not feel well, I have to try harder or make more lifestyle changes.
16.	When my body tells me it needs rest, I do not take the time to provide that.

0 or below 3 items circled: Are you the Buddha? No, seriously. Congratulations to your mental strengths and ability to accept reality as it is. This will save you a lot of energy, that you can direct to where you want to spend it. If you still want to improve your skills, you are welcome to read the chapter on acceptance.

3 items or above circled: We are used and trained to putting up a fight against anything in our life that does not go as planned. A disease is the hallmark of things not going as planned, as no one puts in their calendar: "14th of October: Plan to be admitted to hospital for not feeling mentally well". When we get sick, we have many reasons to accept our current situation. Because in the end, it might help you heal. If you accept your symptoms and do not fight them, you can become clearer on what you can do to ease them. Another thing is that even if symptoms do not clear up, you will have more space to enjoy what is good in your life. Being thankful every day for what you have is an enormous accomplishment and something to be proud of. Get started on your journey to acceptance by reading the dedicated chapter.

Help: I need to improve so much and do not know where to begin

Diseases are often multi factorial and that is why you may miss several root causes of health. Your body can handle quite a lot of imbalance, but somewhere along the line, it all gets too much. That is when we see, for example, the debut of Graves'.

Take a moment to be grateful to your body for managing so well without the attention it needs. It might not be possible for you to change everything at once. Go through them all, one by one.

Another approach is to read about all the root causes of health and choose one that appeals to you. Maybe you have always wanted to try yoga or a gluten-free diet? Fine, that is where you should begin. After a while you will be pumped to implement more improvements to your lifestyle. The root causes of health we often miss are balancing brain and nervous system and restoring adrenals. We are ambitious and do not want to let anybody down. Now, you may skip this if otherwise you will do nothing. Have in mind, though, that leading a stress-free life is a major win for your health. Keep ignoring them and they will come back to bite you.

How to implement habit changes

You know what you have to do - but you are still banging your head against the wall wondering why you do not do it. That happens too many of us, the knowledge is there but motivation is gone fishing.

This is something that is not discussed enough Information alone will not help you change your habits, that is a more complex process and you need to honour that.

Before any lifestyle change, researchers suggest you ask yourself three questions:

On a scale from 1 to 10 - how ready am I to make this change?

If you score 6 or lower, move on to the next question. If you cannot get your score up, choose another goal for yourself. It is important that you do not lie to yourself and say you will make changes that you do not do. This will make you believe less in your word next time, and if you fail yourself again the vicious cycle of "I will begin on Monday" is on.

If you feel powerless or not sure how you will manage this, start small and build from there. Health coaches can be great resources if you need support.

What is important to you about this change?

Image the benefits making this change will have on your life. More energy may mean more play with children and grandchildren. Mental focus may mean you dare to take a class on a subject you have always been interested in. Paint a picture of what life could look like. Focus on the internal benefits rather than the external. Such as, taking a class for your personal development rather than getting ahead in your career and earning more money.

If you want help to find your true motivation, ask yourself this:

- How am I being affected by X (insert root cause of health, for example exercise)?
- What would I most like to change?
- Why am I really concerned about X?
- Is it because of current symptoms or avoiding symptoms in the future? What would my life look like if I did not have to worry about this lifestyle factor?
- What part of me wants to change, and what part does not?
- What is most valuable to me?
- How would this change affect those who are dear to me?

Now you should have an idea about your motivations, see if you get a higher score on the first question.

On a scale of 1 to 10, how certain are you that you can make this change? If the answer is 6 or below, you need to set a smaller goal so it feels attainable. There is nothing wrong with big goals, but you need to see yourself meeting them. Think about a time when you accomplished a health goal.

Small change in mindset - big results

Do you know which habits are helping you and which are hurting you? Make a list of your habits and decide which are useful for meeting you long term goals.

Place your habit in your environment. Want to eat more vegetables? Have a big plate with fresh, attractive veggies on your kitchen counter. Want to meditate more? Read a book on the subject. Also remove objects – unhealthy food, DVDs – that distract you from your habits.

Avoid immediate pleasure. The faster a brain reward comes for a behaviour, the more skeptical you should be. Compare spending time on Facebook versus taking a walk.

Use the 2-minute rule. At the beginning of a new habit, make sure it takes less than 2 minutes to do. Want to being a habit of a daily lunch break walk? The first few times put on your shoes and step outside. Done. This will help you build a foundation of a new habit.

Practice the 2-minute rule. The 2-minute rule is this: when you start a new habit, make sure it takes less than two minutes to do. If your goal is running a marathon, try just tying up your shoes for a couple of minutes. If your habit is to work out at the gym, show up at the gym, and work out for just two minutes. This way, you have a framework that you can actually build upon in developing your habits later on, instead of trying to wish habits into existence.

Build your identity – not your goals. If you see yourself as someone living a healthy life, chances are this will become true. Start building your identity by visiting the sections of the food store that carry veggies and fresh produce. Try cooking the vegetables each week. Talk with friends about their strategies and how they stay healthy. Read about health and use every new habit to form a new identity.

If you get going and stumble somewhere along the way: Do not look back for a second. Brush yourself off and go at it again. Connect with other people who lead healthy lifestyles and if you want, use a health coach who can cheer you on.

CHAPTER 10

CALM IMMUNE SYSTEM

What factors can we influence to improve chances of becoming cured?

Most people agree that lifestyle factors can cause disease. Take smoking or being inactive as examples. Who is arguing that these can make us feel bad and in worst case diagnosed with disease? However, there is resistance to accepting the idea that a positive lifestyle can cure illness. Or what is your opinion if someone claims that exercise can make depression lift, or a gluten-free diet can heal the immune system? We usually ensure that we receive medical treatment for our symptoms. It can often save lives and be invaluable. The enormous advantage of using lifestyle as a complement to healthcare is that you can prevent lots of ill health at once. You do not have to choose between lowering blood pressure, reducing autoimmunity or preventing cancer. You get it all in one package. You must not forget what you can do for your own health. That would give up the power over it and that you should hold on tightly to.

The research available on Graves' tells us that there are several factors you can influence to get cured:

- Choose not to get pregnant
- Be smoke-free
- Reduce stress
- Avoid high iodine intake
- Have adequate vitamin D levels
- Make sure you get enough selenium

- Move and be physically active
- Reduce inflammation.

Stress and recovery

As much as we can, we should avoid stress, but we do not control everything that happens in our lives. Studies suggest that our ability to manage stress seems to be related to how the disease develops. Especially if a patient cannot handle grief and loss, the disease can worsen. If a solution to life's challenges can be found, there is an opportunity to get better. Researchers have also x-rayed the thyroid gland in women with high production of thyroid hormone and seen that it has risen and fallen according to with how stressful life has been.

Women who reported a stressful everyday life 6 months after diagnosis, had a greater risk after 12 months of still having an overactive thyroid gland. The same researchers also found that certain genes could be linked to the risk that stress would affect the course of the disease. But did the women have a stressful everyday life because they had a more active illness, or was it stress that led to worsening illness? We do not know this, but the disease has a major impact on our ability to manage stress. This may show that the disease can cause the experience of stress. The connection to negative life events and the risk of getting the disease suggests that stress triggers the disease. Most likely, there is an interaction between stress and illness - where one leads to the other.

Vitamin D

Research on vitamin D deficiency and autoimmunity shows one difficulty with so-called observational studies. An observational study looks at the relationship between two variables, say vitamin D and Graves'. Then it may turn out, as is also the case with Graves', that patients' levels are deficient. The tricky thing about vitamin D is that you rarely know if the deficiency causes the disease or if the disease is causing the deficiency. Reduced uptake of vitamin D or decreased time outdoors can be two ways the disease could contribute to lower levels. In addition, the status of vitamin D, is probably a marker for good health in general. Those who are young, have normal body weight, eat healthy and exercise - are more likely to have normal vitamin D levels but also a lower risk of chronic disease. Separating the effects of a healthy lifestyle from vitamin D status is therefore difficult. There are diseases where it is completely established that low vitamin D levels are a cause of the disease breaking out. Multiple sclerosis is one example.

Vitamin D has a significant effect on our immune system. Vitamin deficiency has been shown to play a role in more and more conditions of ill health, including autoimmune diseases. Graves' is no exception and vitamin D deficiency can be a contributing factor to illness.

In animal studies with mice, the amount of vitamin D in the diet affect the amount of immune reaction to the TSH receptor. The vitamin can also calm the inflammatory response in both thyroid cells and immune cells.

When Graves' patients with low levels of vitamin D took supplements, the risk of relapse reduced even if it was not possible to show a statistical difference between patients receiving supplements compared with those who did not. However, the time to relapse was significantly delayed. The vitamin D level the study was considered normal if it followed the current guidelines of 50 nmol/l in the blood, but many believe that it is too low for optimal effect. Instead, many researchers say that we should have at least 75 nmol/l of Vitamin D. Ideally 100 to 150 nmol/l. What would have happened if the patients had received supplements up to these levels? Even the researchers themselves wondered if that could provide additional power and want to do studies with higher doses of vitamin D. The vitamin is partly found in the food we eat but the sun is our best source. The vitamin can be formed in the skin when sunlight hits it, but only when the sun is at the right angle. This means that in many regions we only produce our own vitamin D some months of the year. The rest of the year we depend on the body's limited stores in the liver, the diet we eat and supplements. It is easy to check your levels with a blood test. The guidelines for sufficient levels vary, but values from 75 to 150 nmol/l are considered sufficient, 100 to 150 nmol/l optimal.

Selenium

The powerful antioxidant selenium is needed inside the thyroid gland because the production of thyroid hormone is "dirty business". By-products of production are free radicals - strong oxidants that if not taken care of could damage the thyroid gland. Selenium helps one of the cells' most important antioxidants, glutathione, to take care of the free radicals. Selenium also has a role when T4 is to be converted to T3 and can protect the cells against an excess of iodine. Given how important selenium is to the thyroid gland, it may not be surprising that a deficiency shows a link with thyroid disease, including Graves' and even ophthalmopathy.

When the selenium is added to the drug treatment, a faster recovery of TSH and T4 takes place than if selenium was not taken. Other studies have showed that selenium supplements can have a positive effect on quality of life. Patients with active, mild ophthalmopathy may reduce symptoms with selenium supplementation. Much is still unknown about how selenium is best used in Graves'.

A research article summarizes the effects of selenium supplementation in Graves'. Likely positive effects:

- Faster recovery to normal thyroid levels with drug treatment
- Reduces antibodies against the thyroid gland, such as thyroglobulin (but not TRAb)
- Improves symptoms of mild ophthalmopathy and quality of life in some patients.

Possible, but not determined effects:

- Reduces the risk of relapse
- Improves quality of life
- Improves symptoms of moderate or severe ophthalmopathy.

Factors that may affect the effect of supplements:

- Individual selenium levels in the blood
- The level of antibodies
- Form of selenium and dose
- Individual factors such as age, gender, health status, other drugs
- Genetic variations in proteins where selenium is used.

Iodine- healthy supplement or cause of immunity?

The thyroid gland needs about 150 micrograms of iodine per day to produce hormones in sufficient quantities. T4 has four iodine atoms and T3 has, as you might guess, three. In many regions, there are not enough minerals in groundwater and plants for us to get the iodine we need daily. It has previously led to problems with goitre and hypothyroidism. For about 80 years now, some countries have been adding iodine to table salt. This has reduced the problems with goitre not caused by autoimmunity. It is often said that iodine has the potential to trigger Graves' disease. Taking much iodine can trigger Graves' partly because thyroglobulin with more iodine atoms bound to it activates the immune system more easily. Studies have shown that iodine supplementation could cause more relapses in Graves' and in animal studies it has been shown that genetically sensitive individuals become ill with thyroid disease with supplementation. Studies in humans show that in areas where the mineral iodine occurs in sufficient amounts naturally, relapses do not increase. Researchers also believe that the risk of a negative impact of iodine excess mainly arises from selenium deficiency. Many doctors advise to be careful with iodine if you have Graves'. Some advocate a diet low in iodine to cure autoimmune thyroid disease. Avoid supplements of iodine and algae and seaweed with high levels of iodine. However, these have good nutritional values and there are algae that do not naturally absorb iodine, such as spirulina. However, if they are grown with iodine-rich water, they absorb the mineral which is why it is best to check with the manufacturer how it is grown. Also, make sure you have adequate levels of selenium.

Physical activity and recovery

A group of Graves' patients who were encouraged to be physically active for three weeks could end their treatment earlier and reduce the risk of relapse. More about physical activity can be found in the chapter on muscle and bone.

Th2 imbalance in Graves'

The control of immune responses is done by T cells. They can help and regulate other parts of the immune system. Normally they should prevent the body's own tissues from being attacked, but often it does not work. The imbalance in the immune system can differ between different autoimmune diseases. For most autoimmune diseases, it can be established which type of two T-helper cells is dominant in the disease: Th1 or Th2. Th1 dominance leads to more T-cell activity, and Th2 dominance leads to B-cells becoming more active. In Graves', it has been seen that Th2 dominates and another T-helper cell, Th17 cells, forms more pro-inflammatory mediators and that T-regulatory cells cannot calm the immune system as they should. There are normally some immune cells in the thyroid gland, but these are in Graves' abnormally active.

Balancing Th1/Th2 cells is not something that is used in the conventional care of Graves' and there is no research that suggests that it would help to do so. However, there is research on what can tip the scale in favour of one or the other T-cell. Examples of what can shift Th2 to Th1:

- Plant sterols, fat similar to our cholesterol, can increase Th1. Plant sterols are found in plants with fats in them such as avocados, seeds, nuts, and oils.
- Probiotics. Keep an eye out for what bacteria are included in the supplement to promote Th1 or Th2. In traumatic brain injury, the immune system shifts to Th2 dominance, which in one study could be balanced with the help of supplements of lactobacilli: casei, plantarum, acidophilus and delbrueckii bulgaricus; bifidobacteria: breve, longum, and infantis; streptococcus salivarius thermophilus. Lactobacilli inhibit Th2, and the species plantarum is something you can create yourself at home in the kitchen by fermenting vegetables. If you make sauerkraut or kimchi, you also get sulphur-containing vegetables, which can also improve the Th1/Th2 balance. Lactobacillus plantarum that was isolated from kimchi could in studies with human cells suppress immune system overreaction.
- Zinc helps Th1 and supplements could increase the activity of Th1 cells in children with pneumonia and help them recover faster.
- Omega-3 can balance Th1/Th2 without specifically promoting one or the other.
- Medicinal Mushrooms, such as Maitake, Resihi, Cordyceps, turkey tail and Agarcius stimulate Th1.
- Glutamine can strengthen Th1 cells and this amino acid is deficient in Graves'.

Examples of factors that can increase Th2:

- In animal studies, selenium has been shown to increase Th2 activity. As you know, selenium is important in Graves' but make sure you do not exceed the recommended doses.
- Progesterone and melatonin can increase Th2, but the human body makes these hormones naturally, so it is only relevant to consider if you supplement with these.

This was just scratching the surface. If you read other sources about balancing Th1/Th2 - remember that many articles are about results where cells or animals have been used. The effects are often not studied in humans. It is often not yet shown that it is useful for affecting health, including Graves'.

Reduce endocrine disruptors and heavy metals

There are several reasons to reduce your exposure to endocrine disruptors and heavy metals. When you stop consuming them, it can calm the immune system and their presence in nature is reduced. Prevent them entering your body:

- Avoid buying and using plastic items. In contact with food and beverages, especially warm and fatty, the hormone-disrupting chemicals from the plastic can move into the food or drink.
- Eat organic so you avoid residues of endocrine disruptors and pesticides in the food.
- Avoid cans, they are often lined with the endocrine disruptor BPA on the inside.
- Remove soft plastic such as yoga mats or gloves. They may contain endocrine disruptors such as phthalates. There are non-toxic options if you keep an eye out.
- Buy make-up and hygiene products with clean ingredients. Unfortunately, the beauty industry has not as clear labels as the food industry, but find brands you trust.
- Choose fish and fish oil caught in as clean water as possible.
- Avoid chemically impregnated wood and opt for an environmentally friendly treatment. Pressure impregnation often contain heavy metals.
- Skip furniture and other items with flame retardant treatments. Sometimes, for example, covers and pyjamas are treated with these endocrine disruptors.

- Remove amalgam fillings if it is found that they leak mercury into the body.

Support detoxification

It can be very scary to think about all the toxins we are exposed to daily. Besides reducing your exposure, you can take the help of your body's own detoxification system when you want to get rid of unwanted toxins.

You have several ways to get rid of toxins: Urine, stool, sweat, and by storing them in hair. Before they can be sent out through these various pathways, the liver needs to prepare the toxins for excretion. Your liver handles dangerous toxins every day so you can get rid of them. Here are some ways you can help your body get rid of toxins:

- Drink enough water. It helps toxins to be cleared out.
- Help your gut produce stool every day. Examples of things that can help: Move, eat fibre and drink water. Stress can cause slower bowel movements.
- Sweat regularly. Shower immediately after a workout or sauna to rinse off what has been excreted.
- Give the liver a lot of nutrition and energy. A nutrient-dense diet in sufficient quantity helps the liver remove toxins, which is an energy- and nutritionally demanding process.
- Sleep well. During sleep, organs and cells are cleared of waste products. Too little sleep means that the cells do not have enough time to clean themselves.

Glutathione - several potential benefits in Graves'

Glutathione is a fantastic molecule your body itself can produce. It can balance the immune system, increase efficiency of detox pathways, and act as an antioxidant. It has been found that the levels of glutathione in Graves' are low.

There are several potential advantages to increasing your levels of glutathione in Graves':

- Glutathione is included in the enzymes that remove free radicals and thus lowers the inflammation that otherwise can contribute to autoimmunity.
- Decreased levels of glutathione are a factor that can lead to Th2 dominance.
- Glutathione is a powerful antioxidant and can reduce symptoms and speed recovery during the time thyroid hormone levels are high.
- Supports the liver when it is not nourished to maintain detoxification.

Ways to increase your glutathione levels with the help of lifestyle:

- Sufficient selenium intake. Selenium is a cofactor for glutathione and is needed for its function.
- Increased intake of sulphur-containing vegetables such as cabbage and onions. Sulphur is needed to form glutathione. Eggs contain cysteine, which is a sulphur-containing amino acid.
- Vitamin C- rich foods can help increase glutathione levels.
- Sleeping, exercising, and reducing alcohol intake are other ways to increase glutathione.
- The heavy metal mercury depletes our glutathione stores. Mercury can be found in water we drink, food we eat or come from amalgam fillings in the teeth

Glutathione supplementation can be a help right at the time of diagnosis when the body is most vulnerable to oxidative stress and has the least nutrition available to build glutathione. Glutathione requires the amino acid glutamine to be formed, which is an established deficiency in diagnosis. To support production, you can choose to either take the glutamine supplements or taking glutathione directly. Vitamin C and N-Acetylcysteine (NAC) can also help form glutathione. If you choose supplementation of glutathione, choose a so-called liposomal variant. There, the glutathione is encapsulated in fat, which facilitates absorption in the intestine and its delivery to the cells where it is needed.

Reverse biological age

There is not much to do about getting chronologically older. Older age is also associated with increased risk of chronic diseases, Graves' included. But it does not have to be this way. Nobel Prize winner professor Elizabeth Blackburn and health psychologist Elissa Epel write in their book "The telomere effect" about the difference between life span and health span. Two people may die at the same age but one may have been plagued by diseases for a long time and the other has not. The reason, according Blackburn and Epel, is the effect our lifestyle has on our DNA. Our telomeres that are the caps at the end that protect our DNA strands. They work like the plastic caps on shoelaces and when they break up the lace withers. Same with our DNA and the cell inevitably ages - and you with it.

What gives great hope are all the things you can do to reduce your biological age and protect your telomeres:

- Your telomeres listen to your thoughts so make sure you have a positive inner dialogue.

- Mind-body techniques have a profound impact on us. Use the meditation discovered by Blackburn to have a positive effect on telomeres - Kirtan Kriya. Search on YouTube for a guided videos on how to do it.
- Make sure you move your body. You may feel younger immediately and cellularly it is true as your telomeres lengthen.
- Seek the company of supportive and loving people. Humans are pack animals, and we thrive together. If you feel lonely or do not have time to see friends or family, make it a priority. Your age depends on it.

CHAPTER 11

NOURISHED BY DIET AND SUPPLEMENTS

Ann-Louise's story: I used diet as a tool to recover after Graves'

"I was diagnosed with Graves' in 2009 and treated with block and replace. In 2012, the disease returned, then my thyroid was irradiated and I have been taking Levothyroxine ever since. Since the radiation, I have felt worse every year, but it can also be because of tough years as a new mom. In the autumn of 2019, my iron levels were low. I then started eating iron tablets and feel much better, but I guess I will always have to struggle with nutritional deficiencies. I have read about anti-inflammatory diet and from what I understand, my diet may have triggered the disease, partly because I have eaten too much inflammatory foods in my life. I feel better when I eat anti-inflammatory in the form of a paleo diet. With an anti-inflammatory diet, I do not have as much pain in my body and I become more flexible, less stiff. I feel young again. The most important difference is that I become as alert and normal as I used to be. I feel that grains are the worst, I get exhausted and almost paralyzed, have difficulties grabbing things and feel mentally unwell. However, sometimes I do not stay away from bread and similar foods. Therefore, my health goes up and down. I also have normal stools when I exclude sugar, milk products and grains. I have never experienced this before in my life, the normal thing for me has always been to have loose stools and having to rush to the toilet."

*

Diet as a tool for increased quality of life

"We humans have always known the following miracle: Food gives us energy, and it heals and repairs our bodies. With every bite we take, we have the opportunity to either create health or increase the risk of disease."

Mark Hyman, functional medicine physician and author

When we use the power of the diet's impact on health and quality of life, we have three goals: replenish nutrition, improve the intestinal flora and reduce inflammation. Our tools for getting there are to add everything we can of food that benefits these goals and remove food that prevents us from getting there. Impaired intestinal flora can cause increased inflammation and inflammation can cause a deteriorated intestinal flora. It can be a vicious cycle. When we heal ourselves, we also need nutrients to rebuild the body, something that is not abundant in Graves'.

Reload on nutrition

A high-speed metabolism consumes more nutrients. Nutrients that are needed to keep inflammation and the immune system in check. It is a huge stress for the body to maintain energy production, and other processes at a higher rate. Therefore, it is not surprising that lacking several nutrients is common in Graves'. Among them are iron, selenium, zinc, all of which are important for a normally functioning thyroid gland. Other common nutritional deficiencies in patients with Graves': amino acids (building blocks of proteins), vitamins (A, B6, B5, B1, C and D) and minerals (phosphorus, magnesium, potassium, sodium, chromium). Besides the high metabolism using more of our nutrients, they can occur when biochemical processes become disrupted, which leads to higher or lower production or consumption of some nutrients.

Antioxidants are lacking when we have high thyroid hormones and for one of the most important, CoQ10, the levels are among the lowest measured in humans. Vitamin E is a protector of the fats in the body. Selenium is also an important antioxidant and, as we have seen before, plays a major role in protection against oxidative stress. When levels drop, as they do in Graves', tissues and cells more readily oxidize, which can contribute too many of our most common public health diseases.

The brain, muscles and heart are also depleted of nutrients they need for their function. Myo-inositol is a carbohydrate with effects on the neurotransmitter serotonin and plays a role in the risk of depression. When researchers measured levels of nutrients in the brain of patients with Graves', myo-inositol was significantly lower. Also, choline important for some of the most basic functions of the brain such as keeping the cell walls intact, had lower levels. Choline is also a precursor to the neurotransmitter acetylcholine, the parasympathetic nervous system's most important neurotransmitter. Acetylcholine can promote memory and people whose diet contains a lot of choline have higher chances of better memory. Choline and myo-inositol levels seem to recover in most patients, after restored thyroid hormone levels. But there are other nutrients, important for the brain, that do not seem to do so: glutamine and glutamate. Glutamine is a neurotransmitter in the brain and also a precursor of another neurotransmitter - glutamate. The pattern of low glutamine and glutamate has also been seen in patients with depression. Higher T3 led to greater imbalances of these neurotransmitters in the brain.

Muscles also depend on the right nutrients to do their job and Graves' has been shown to reduce one of the most important ones - carnitine. Carnitine is found in high concentration in muscles and heart. It is crucial for energy production and it can transport away accumulated waste products. When we with Graves' consume our body's supply of carnitine, it can lead to energy production not working optimally. But not only that, reduced carnitine also causes the cells to lose protection from high levels of thyroid hormone. Both T4 and T3 can be blocked by carnitine from entering the cell nucleus, which reduces the negative effects of excess hormones. Because of these effects, researchers believe that it may be reasonable to supplement carnitine to patients with Graves' disease. Patients with Graves' who received 990 mg carnitine twice daily also experienced reduced fatigue and some patients also experienced reduced mental fatigue. Carnitine is also found in the brain and when we get too low levels, it can affect the nerve cells' ability to function normally by reducing energy production, increasing oxidative stress and even causing cell death.

Can antioxidants be a complement to other treatment?

Researchers believe that it is likely that the oxidative stress during the disease causes some problems of the we experience in Graves'. Therefore, it is not far off to investigate treatment with antioxidants. Some studies have tested vitamin C, propolis, vitamin E and other antioxidants besides the usual drug treatment.

The first study with antioxidants tested vitamin C at 1000 mg/day besides drug treatment for a month. This improved the antioxidant defense system and reduced oxidative stress. Other studies have since expanded these initial results. In one of these later studies, 56 patients took part and were divided into three groups. The study lasted for two months:

Group 1: Drug treatment only

Group 2: A mixture of antioxidants (vitamin E, beta carotene, vitamin C, copper, zinc, magnesium, and selenium) only

Group 3: Combination of drugs and antioxidants

The doctors noted thyroid status, oxidative stress and symptoms of the disease. Group 1 had normalized thyroid values, reduced oxidative stress and fewer symptoms. Group 2 still had elevated hormone levels but decreased oxidative stress and fewer symptoms. The last group, group 3, had faster normalization of thyroid levels and faster reduction of symptoms than the other two groups.

Besides the antioxidants mentioned above, there are further studies with propolis and CoQ10. Propolis is the putty in hives and contains hundreds of nutrients, including many antioxidants. Here, experimental rats and not people with hyperthyroidism and oxidative stress were examined. 10 micrograms of propolis/kg or lb of body weight sufficed to protect the rats from oxidative stress. Researchers believe that propolis works in three different ways to protect against oxidative stress: neutralizes free radicals, reduces oxidation of fat, and increases antioxidant status. CoQ10 has been studied in patients with hyperthyroidism, and one study showed that 120 mg/day for one week improved heart function. If you are being treated with beta blockers, you should also know these reduce your own production of CoQ10. The production of Q10 also decreases with age. A study in which Graves' patients deficient in Q10 received a supplement of 30 mg/day for two years had improved normalization of the thyroid tissue.

Is it a good idea to add antioxidants to my medication?

Yes, some researchers believe that antioxidants besides drug treatment early in diagnosis can be beneficial to patients through faster control of the disease, thanks to the recovery of hormone levels and symptoms.

Ophthalmopathy and antioxidants

Free radicals play a fundamental role in the development of eye disease, and it is probably the ability of cigarette smoke to create oxidative stress that is the link to why smokers have an increased risk.

Small studies with cells from patients with Graves' ophthalmopathy have shown positive effects of treatment with antioxidants such as N-Acetylcysteine, vitamin C and vitamin B3. Selenium has also been studied and there is probably a benefit to using this antioxidant in mild eye disease. It is encouraging that we might get help of supplements with antioxidants, but we must keep in mind that the cause of oxidative stress, in this case an activated immune system, is the most important to overcome.

Antioxidant supplements no lifelong miracle cure

For a long time, antioxidant supplements have been marketed as preventing aging and disease. Obviously, they can be helpful in conditions where the production of free radicals is uncontrolled, but there is not much to suggest that you benefit from taking them for a long time. Rather, supplements of vitamin E, vitamin A and beta-carotene in high doses have been linked to the risk of dying prematurely. Why is that? One reason is that these supplements reduce the body's production of its own antioxidants and these are more important to take care of free radicals and prevent ill health linked to them. In Graves', the body does not have time to form its own antioxidants, and supplements can therefore provide support until its own levels are restored. The studies on Graves' patients and antioxidants have used supplements for eight weeks and early after diagnosis. Selenium and CoQ10 are the exceptions that confirm the rule. You may benefit from their protective effects in thyroid disease and take them as a supplement for a longer period beyond the initial time of diagnosis. The longest study was nine months long and researchers could then still see positive effects. The effects of selenium in Graves' may be due to the fact that it is included in enzymes that are part of the body's own antioxidant defenses and enzymes that protect against excess iodine.

That said, antioxidants are still an important key to health - but it should be your own antioxidants or those that occur naturally in the diet. One reason exercise has health benefits is that it leads to the cells forming more of their own antioxidants. The same applies to fasting, sunlight and phytonutrients found in vegetables.

Interview with Karl Hultén, Master of Biomedicine: Restoring nutritional deficiencies

Karl Hultén is one founder of Paleoteket, whose goal is to help people take control of their own health. Karl is an expert on diet and lifestyle in autoimmune disease. He has a master's degree in biomedicine, has autoimmune disease himself and has used the autoimmune protocol, AIP to become virtually symptom free. He began helping others in 2009. Today he focuses on online trainings on AIP, paleo diet and functional medicine. He has a podcast on autoimmune health and has written several books.

What does it take to restore nutritional deficiencies?

"The most common deficiencies I see among those with autoimmune diseases differ little from the general population. The most common, and this is also true globally, is iron deficiency. Something common in the population but even more common among those with autoimmune is vitamin D deficiency. Vitamin B12 deficiency is not as common in the population but common in autoimmune disease. Magnesium deficiency is also common in the public and people with autoimmune disease."

Karl Hultén says that your nutritional status is determined by three things:

- Eating habits

- Gut health
- Lifestyle

He explains that your nutritional deficiencies reflect our eating habits.

"With a simple blood test, I can see if a person is vegan, vegetarian, or just eating small amount of meat. They often have deficiency of iron and/or B12. If they eat a smaller proportion of vegetables, they are more often deficient in magnesium and potassium". How to restore nutritional habits is individual but most effective according to Karl is to improve diet and gut health. But other lifestyle factors also come into play.

"For the absolute majority, it is enough to change the diet to address nutritional deficiencies. A paleo diet with meat, fish, poultry, vegetables, root vegetables, nuts and seeds and leafy vegetables is estimated to contain 200 to 300 percent of the daily requirement of all essential nutrients. For most people, it is enough to switch to a paleo diet with whole ingredients to correct nutritional deficiencies and regain their gut health".

For a good nutritional balance, you also need to think about what you do not eat:

"It is not just about filling the nutritional needs, but also about not triggering poor gut health. The food must contain the essential nutrients to replenish levels. But even if the diet is complete, you cannot eat things you are sensitive to, because then local inflammation is created in the gut, which reduces the absorption of nutrients. A clear sign of this is B12 deficiency. But anything that can trigger poor gut health can cause nutritional deficiencies.

Common foods that can do this are mainly grains or other foods with lectins, foods that irritate the intestinal wall, various food additives, sugar and processed foods. If you remove these and replace them with whole foods, many reached an improved gut health. For the remaining, it is usually about working individually improving gut health and in other cases to take the health of a functional medical practitioner."

What can impair nutrient uptake?

Karl gives a list of situations that can impair nutrient uptake:

Foods with a negative impact on gut health such as grains that include lectins, like gluten.

Dysbiosis, imbalance in the intestinal flora as overgrowth of bacteria in the small intestine (SIBO).

Infections, by parasites or bacteria.

Medicines, such as antacids.

"These factors can affect the intestinal mucosa so it cannot absorb nutrients efficiently. This can cause malnutrition, and systemic inflammation. Bacteria can enter the body and trigger the immune system to immune reactions against its own tissues. Then autoimmune disease occurs. If you in addition have nutritional deficiencies, it will contribute to impairing the immune system's function."

Karl Hultén explains it as a vicious circle where the wrong diet reduces the uptake of nutrients but it also stresses the body and the immune system so that consumption of some nutrients increases.

The CoQ10 deficiency in Graves' is an example where increased metabolism results from the increased consumption of oxygen and free radical formation. Then the need for CoQ10 increases so much that stocks run out. That is how inflammatory processes can consume nutrients and in this case also enzymes important for the body".

Obstacles when we want to restore nutrition

Karl explains which are the most common obstacles that can appear when we want to restore nutritional balance.

"Often people have too low consumption of animal foods, mainly red meat. Excessive consumption of foods that trigger bad gut health is also common. In other cases, it may be age that makes it more difficult. Older people eat less and have a slight iron and B12 deficiency, and they also take more drugs that may interact with nutrients or consume them. If you have already switched to a diet with whole foods, the cause of not restoring nutrient levels might be a food sensitivity to, for example, eggs or potato. Last, there may be an infection or dysbiosis behind it."

Anyone who eats a one-sided keto diet or carnivore diet may be at risk of magnesium deficiency.

"Many people experience that extra magnesium, is relaxing and facilitates sleep. However, I am not sure how worried we should be about magnesium deficiency in an evolutionary diet. In the population, magnesium deficiency is linked to poor bone health, cardiovascular disease, metabolic syndrome and type-2 diabetes. But these are remedied with paleo diet, type 2 diabetes reverses in basically two weeks. It is uncertain how accurate the reference range for magnesium in blood samples is because they refer to people who eat a high-grain diet."

Karl Hultén usually recommends the addition of magnesium. He believes that 400 mg per day, sometimes more than that, is sufficient because the body gets rid of the excess via urine and regulates absorption in the intestine.

Increase nutrition with diet

Karl gives three examples of recovery of nutritional deficiencies:

Iron deficiency. A large proportion of girls have iron deficiency, mainly due to the fact that they eat too little meat. Most of our severe nutritional deficiencies are due to the fact that we eat too few animal foods. When we eat little meat, we instead have to cover our needs from plants where nutrients are often not found in their most easily absorbed forms. Iron, for example, is found in plants in an ionic form that we only absorb a little of, unlike the haem form in meat, which we absorb much more easily. By increasing the intake of animal foods, you can fix iron deficiency in a few weeks.

Vitamin D deficiency is common in the population and most young women. It depends partly on the diet and also on our exposure to sun light. We spend too much time indoors and use, after spending the winter inside, sunscreen that prevents vitamin D from forming in the skin.

B-12 is found mainly in seafood and offal, but also meat and eggs. B-12 is one of the most difficult nutritional deficiencies to address and can persist even in people who eat enough of the vitamin. This is because the uptake of B12 is a sensitive multi-step process. Components in saliva interact with what is called intrinsic factor that is formed in the gut. The complex must then reach the small intestine where it is activated and taken up by specific receptors in the intestinal wall. The process can be disrupted by many things: imbalance in the intestinal flora so that the receptors are not expressed and taking antacids reduces the formation of intrinsic factor because it requires hydrochloric acid. Alcohol abuse can also reduce intrinsic factor and autoimmune diseases that attack the cells that secrete intrinsic factor. Therefore, it is not always enough to take the daily requirement of B12, but you may need to review all these factors."

*

Some of our most nutritious foods

A nutrient-dense diet is a prerequisite for returning all the nutrients the body has consumed.

Offal. Liver is one of nature's multivitamin and mineral supplements. It is the most nutritious food you can eat. Liver contains many of the nutrients low in Graves': carnitine, choline, cholesterol, vitamins and minerals, but also the antioxidants CoQ10 and Alpha Lipoic Acid (ALA). Contrary to many people's beliefs, the liver is not a place where the body stores toxins. These are sent out with urine and stool or stored in our adipose tissue. The liver pâté you buy in the food store is unfortunately deprived of much of the nutrition and is not recommended. Make your own instead.

Seafood. Oysters are a source of many nutrients, especially those essential for the thyroid. Fatty fish are an excellent source of omega-3 fatty acids. Sea food and fish are also a source of iodine, which some believe people with Graves' should be careful with. Eat them but avoid in daily xcessive amounts.

Egg yolk. Another one of nature's multivitamin and mineral supplements. The yellow is more nutritious and often called a "brain food". The white contains less nutrition but more high-quality proteins.

Meat. Eating or not eating meat can be debated, but here we are talking nutritious food and meat is a good source of nutrition. If you want to choose more climate-friendly meat, buy grass-fed meat or even better wild caught. Offal and poultry also have lower climate footprints.

Nuts and seeds. Full of fibre, minerals, fat and carbohydrates makes the energy from these last longer. Those who regularly eat nuts live healthier and longer. Selenium is especially abundant in Brazil nuts, 2 per day can cover your daily needs. However, the amount of selenium in nuts can vary, which is why you who want to be on the safe side with dosing should choose supplements. Nuts and seeds are relatively high in omega-6 - fatty acids, while walnuts, chia seeds and flaxseed contain more omega-3. Omega-6 is associated with inflammation and you need to keep the ratio between the omegas in mind. A ratio of between 1:4 and 4:1 is considered healthy, but a western diet often contains 15:1 or more of omega-6 to omega-3 which will drive inflammation.

Vegetables. Peppers, onions, cruciferous plants such as kale, broccoli and cabbage, carrots and spinach are vegetables with extra nutritional value. Seaweed and algae, such as spirulina and chlorella, are also nutritious. Spirulina may contain iodine, depending on how it is grown. Chlorella contains moderate amounts of iodine, but also here levels can vary. Ask the manufacturer if you want to be sure. Vegetables with a high liquid content, cucumbers and radishes have a poorer nutrient content.

A real goldmine are our wild vegetables and mushrooms, they are packed with nutrients and good for our climate. Nettles top the list, but also dandelion are some of the most nutritious vegetables you can eat. Wild plants are tougher than our cultivated ones and the same plant chemicals they use to strengthen themselves against attacks from insects, weather, and wind also benefit our health. The toughness is reflected in the taste, which some think is challenging, but a handful of nettles in a smooth soup or dandelion leaves in a salad are nice culinary additions. A bonus is that you also get fibre your gut bacteria will love. Inulin, a fibre in dandelion, is considered a superfood for good bacteria. Wild plants are also free, and you get to enjoy nature when you pick them.

People who eat predominantly vegetables in their diet also have a lower risk of developing Graves'. Vegans and vegetarians had the lowest risk, people who also ate fish and eggs medium risk and carnivores the highest risk. The study is a so-called observational study, and it is therefore difficult to know if someone got Graves' less often because they otherwise lived healthier or if it was the vegetables, or the absence of the meat, that was the key to the reduced risk. In their study, the researchers discuss several reasons a diet high in vegetables can protect against Graves':

- Vegans and vegetarians have lower body weight, which reduces the risk of autoimmunity.
- They also have lower levels of insulin-like growth factor-1 (IGF-1) which can affect the immune system.
- Plant chemicals in vegetables such as polyphenols, flavonoids and antioxidants can protect against autoimmunity.
- In meat, there may be endocrine disruptors with potential effects on hormone balance and autoimmunity.

Eat plenty of vegetables - at least 500 grams, preferably 800 grams per day. To reach these levels, it is usually required that you eat vegetables at every meal, including breakfast. Choose your meat carefully and do not eat more than you need for nutrition and protein.

Herbs and spices. As with our wild vegetables, the strong taste suggests that these are real tough plants. That means nutritious food for us. Be generous with spices and herbs in your food. Your taste buds will also thank you.

Cocoa. Fat, carbohydrates and protein. These are found in cocoa. Nutrients that plants contribute are called phytonutrients and cocoa is packed with them. Choose chocolate with 90 percent or 100 cocoa content or make your own chocolate without added sugar. Cocoa called "raw", that is - not roasted, can contain larger amounts of phytonutrients.

About nutrition for the brain

The brain is a major consumer of energy and nutrition. To keep it healthy and help it recover, we should eat nutritiously. Some groups of nutrients are especially important for the brain.

In a separate category of nutrients, but just as important as vitamins and minerals, we find the phytonutrients. These give plants their colours and flavours. Each colour comes from a unique plant chemical. The carrot and pumpkin have their carotenoids, the tomato and watermelon their lycopene and so on. An important health advice is therefore that you should "eat the rainbow", preferably every day. In future chapters the importance of supporting the brain with your lifestyle will be clarified. Then think back to the phytonutrients - or a subset of them - polyphenols.

Take advantage polyphenol power

Polyphenols are antioxidants and feed your good gut bacteria. Benefits of polyphenols:

- Reduced inflammation
- Lower blood pressure
- Slower aging
- Blood glucose control
- Better cardiovascular health
- Positive for the intestinal flora
- Strengthens brain health.

If we pause at that last thing: strengthen brain health. Improved brain function and prevention of serious diseases that affect the brain, such as Alzheimer's, may result from increased content of polyphenols in the diet. They can increase blood flow in the brain, the formation of new nerve cells and the brain's ability to adapt and improve, but also inhibit activity of harmful processes in the brain. Just as polyphenols are positive for heart health because they are anti-inflammatory, they are thought to do the same for the brain. Even low blood pressure, good blood flow along with good blood sugar control are linked to a healthy brain. 150 mg of cocoa polyphenols in healthy volunteers could increase blood flow to the brain and a single large dose of at least 520 mg of polyphenols (again from cocoa) could improve performance on brain function tests. Other particularly rich sources of polyphenols are turmeric, green and black tea, berries, coffee and nuts such as pecans and hazelnuts. Spices and herbs also contain large amounts of polyphenols.

Put coffee on hold

Coffee is a rich source of polyphenols, and many of us love to drink it. When you cure your Graves' disease, it is still a good idea to pause coffee. This is because coffee places demand on the adrenal glands and nervous system. Coffee adds no energy - it instead triggers the body's stress response to chase it out. In the long run, we can get more tired if we drink coffee. Many also testify that they no longer tolerate coffee as well in Graves'. Also try to skip cocoa, tea and other stimulants if you feel you need it. Cutting coffee might mean that your biggest source of antioxidants disappears, as many in the west get a substantial amount of antioxidants from their java. Do not let that happen because these are essential to health. Find other ways to get your polyphenols, choose from the list above, but also consider pausing cocoa and tea that are not herbal as some may be sensitive to those too.

Healthy fats for the brain

For a long time, fat has been what health-conscious people have avoided more than anything else. New ideas are questioning this, and the role of fat has been restored to be an important part of a healthy diet. The dry mass of your brain is made up of two-thirds of fat - largely omega-3 and phosphatidylserine. They can be found in the cell wall of every nerve cell and the fat is also the insulation around the protrusions the nerve cells use to communicate with each other. To eat good fats is to take care of your brain, it is needed for it to function optimally. Eat, for example: good quality oils, fatty seafood, coconut, meat from wild or grass-grazing animals, olives, nuts and seeds, avocados, butter or ghee. Other nutrients for the brain:

Carnitine, cholesterol, ALA and CoQ10 preferably in combination with B vitamins. Found in liver but also in foods from the sea such as sardines, oysters, and mussels.

Healthy gut reduces inflammation

The gastrointestinal tract is the largest surface we have exposed to the outside world, it is larger than the skin. The entire digestive system is about seven meters long. Technically, the intestine is still part of the outside and therefore the body needs to be very attentive to what is happening there. The barrier between inside and outside is only a single cell layer thick. Therefore, it is not surprising that two thirds of our immune cells are located in and around our gastrointestinal tract. The gut must maintain a balance between keeping intruders out and letting in nutrients and water. The immune cells help maintain this balance. The gut is a training camp for our immune system and the contents of the gastrointestinal tract, including the food and bacteria in the gut flora, are the personal trainers. They teach the immune cells how to react, and what to react to. The bacteria in the gut have several ways they communicate with the immune system to tell that they are friend or foe. For a healthy intestinal flora, a large variety of bacteria and an intestinal mucosa in good shape are needed. The diversity should preferably resemble a rainforest - many species ensure our well-being, while a reduced diversity of intestinal bacteria can cause disease. There are bacteria throughout the gastrointestinal tract. In the mouth, the number is the smallest and then it accumulates along the way until we reach the colon where a small patch contains billions of intestinal bacteria. A lot of the energy consumed at rest is used to keep our mucous membranes (that means intestines, eyes, nose and vagina) intact and free from intruders. Around the intestine is the lymphatic system where many immune cells are located, but many of them are also located directly below the intestinal barrier. The gut and intestinal flora take part in most physiological and immunological processes. The knowledge about how the intestinal flora can affect well-being, gut health, hormone balance, the thyroid gland and more, is increasing every day. The intestinal flora has an important role to play. Your health, both emotionally and physically, is largely determined by your gut flora. Is it healthy and dominated by good bacteria good for you and reduce inflammation? Or has it been taken over by harmful bacteria that promote inflammation? Lipopolysaccharides (LPS) are part of the cell wall of some harmful bacteria. It is good at triggering inflammation and researchers even use it when they want to do experiments where inflammation is to be induced. It is not uncommon for our guts to contain bacteria with this molecule in the cell wall. It can cause inflammation in the intestine or sometimes leak out into the body. The good news is that you can influence the flora with your lifestyle mainly through how many types of fibre from plants you eat. Larger number of fibres = larger number of intestinal bacteria. The body can control the intestinal flora by, for example, signalling via the nervous system. When we feel calm or exercise (not too much though as this is unhealthy for the gut), it sends anti-inflammatory signals to the intestines. It is a constant exchange of information where the intestinal flora affects the body, but the body also affects the intestinal flora.

Your gut flora works hard

Here are some ways in which the intestinal flora contributes to your health:

The immune system. The bacteria's genes signal the immune system around the intestines that control local and systemic inflammation and play a role in whether you develop allergies or autoimmune diseases.

Detox. Residual products from the metabolism are formed in the liver and excreted with the bile to the intestine where they accompany the stool out. The intestinal flora is important in that it can break down toxins (including carcinogens) so they can then be removed from the body.

Vitamin and neurotransmitter production. You depend on the bacteria in your gut to make vitamin K2, vitamin B12, niacin, pyridoxine (B6), serotonin and other nutrients.

Uptake and production of nutrients. Bacteria in our gut can help us break down complex carbohydrates. You could not break down a single fruit or vegetable without their help. We have lived forever in symbiosis with bacteria, and we simply depend on them to do the job. The bacteria can also produce short-chain fatty acids (SCFA), important for our health. They have been shown to increase the intestinal uptake of water, stimulate the formation of new intestinal cells and they may even be part of the defence against type 2 diabetes, inflammatory bowel disease (IBS) and other diseases.

Protection against pathogens. Infections can affect us by leaving unwanted, pathogenic microbes in the gut. Your gut flora can help your immune system fight the uninvited guests. The more and more viable good intestinal bacteria that have established themselves in the gut, the less room for uninvited guests to settle down.

Improve the gut flora

The major way to influence the gut flora is through what you eat. A study of depressed patients had participants either be treated with drugs plus eat a diet adapted to stimulate a healthier gut flora or treated only with drugs. The diet was a Mediterranean diet with slightly less meat than usual but extra virgin olive oil and nuts. After 12 weeks, one third of the diet group did no longer fit the diagnosis criteria of depression.

But gut flora depends not only on diet. The American Gut Project was founded in 2012 by researchers in the field. They want to better understand the human microbiome, all the bacteria we live in symbiosis with. They are curious about which bacteria are present where, how many they are and how they are affected by diet, lifestyle, and disease. In their research, they have made a list of factors for a healthier intestinal flora. The most important factor comes first.

A varied plant-based diet. Fibre from plants + good bacteria = true. If you eat less than 5 different plants a week and instead increase to 30, you get a huge effect on the gut flora. But a little is better than nothing at all. Doubling from five to ten also gives an effect. Invest in eating plants of different colors and from different plant groups. Eat a mix of leafy greens, fruits, berries, legumes, onions and so on.

How old you are. As early as the age of 20, the species richness in the intestine decreases. In addition, the proportion of bacteria with a negative impact on health increases.

Inflammatory bowel disease. Local inflammation in parts of the intestine benefits bacteria linked to ill health. If you have an inflammatory bowel disease, your intestinal flora is therefore disturbed. A disturbed intestinal flora can also cause inflammation in the rest of the intestine and body.

The season. We have a more varied intestinal flora during the summer. We are outside more and there are more fresh vegetables available. The outdoor air contains bacteria and other organisms, as well as plant parts that can all stimulate the intestinal flora. A reason to take a walk in the woods, even in winter.

Antibiotics. A double-edged sword as we have overcome many serious diseases thanks to these drugs. Unfortunately, they not only kill the bad bacteria that infect us but also the good ones. Take antibiotics when you really need them, but consult your doctor if you can avoid it. After a course of antibiotics, it takes time for the intestinal flora to recover and in the worst case, some species of bacteria will never return.

Male or female. There are gender differences between the intestinal flora of men and women. No one knows exactly why, but the sex hormones are suspected to affect this. These differences are sometimes claimed to explain why women suffer more from autoimmune disease. When the hormones fluctuate, as during pregnancy and breastfeeding, so does the intestinal flora.

Sleep. Are you surprised that good sleep is linked to more good bacteria? Probably not. Another reason to make sure you get the rest you need every night.

Obesity. Obesity leaves a negative an impression on our intestinal flora and the connection between BMI and the composition of the gut flora is clear. Obesity causes more proinflammatory bacteria.

Alcohol. Over one to two servings per day adversely affects the gut flora.

Exercise. Those who exercise have a richer intestinal flora. But being balanced about exercise is best. Exercise when you have a disturbed intestinal flora, are not used to exercising or have poor eating habits can affect the intestines negatively. Too much exercise is a stress for the body, and for the intestinal flora.

Interview with Gunilla Saupe, licensed physician: Awaken the power of your self-healing

Gunilla Saupe is a licensed doctor and runs a private clinic north of Stockholm. Gunilla has long been interested in complementary medicine and has taken courses in homeopathy, manual treatments and lifestyle medicine such as diet, physical activity and relaxation. Gunilla has a long experience in the trearment thyroid problems with NDT. Many patients seek her out for alternative treatment for thyroid disease.

Graves' patients usually come to Gunilla after a period of illness, not in the acute stage.

"I usually see Graves' patients when they have undergone radioiodine therapy or surgery and have ended up in hypothyroidism. They may also have had an untreated Graves', and after that slipped into hypothyroidism. Most people who need treatment feel best on natural thyroid extract (NDT). Better than on synthetic alternatives. I see that regardless of whether you had hypothyroidism from the beginning or Graves'. Our bodies can make use of the natural hormones completely differently. It rhymes with our physiology and you get a more effective symptom relief.

Of my patients with hypothyroidism, the largest proportion also have antibodies, TPO antibodies or both TPO and TG. My experience is that with an anti-inflammatory diet, we can affect autoimmunity."

Diet is a great opportunity for all of us to influence our health, says Gunilla. She has seen repeatedly how changing the diet can affect symptoms and reduce autoimmunity.

"Anyone who wants to maintain good health and prevent disease should eat an anti-inflammatory diet. If you also have an established autoimmune disease, there are obvious health reasons to avoid becoming more ill and reduce autoimmunity. An anti-inflammatory diet is to me the most important tool for health. For many years I have known getting healthy is very much about reducing intake of what we know triggers inflammation. This includes gluten - all gluten-containing grains. This includes refined sugar and other refined carbohydrates and dairy products. These are the "white toxins": white flour, white sugar, and milk. If you really want to go all in, which is recommended, it is best to reduce and then exclude all three. Then you get the absolute best results. Of those who do, many find that their gut functions much better. They become less gassy, do not have pain and are not constipated. An unbalanced gut is the basis of most of our diseases, so it is important that we ensure a good gastrointestinal function."

The diet does the most for the one who is sickest

When we are the sickest and most tired, it can be tough to get a grip of your diet, but Gunilla believes that this is when we need it the most.

"The sicker we are, it does not matter what chronic disease we have, the better for the body's self-healing ability that we relieve the body from these foods. I strongly believe that we should see ourselves as self-healing individuals and a self-healing system and use our awareness to make various positive choices to help self-healing in the best way."

The food can also contain chemicals from fertilizers or pesticides. According to Gunilla, to help the body heal, it is better to choose organic foods.

"Eat food made from scratch with organic foods as far as possible to avoid toxins accumulating in our bodies. We need to be aware not to poison our bodies unnecessarily. The toxins are harmful to all organ systems and eventually the scale tips, and we see many symptoms. With good home- cooked food we know what ingredients we put in the food, we can avoid additives that are otherwise found in processed food. We also know today that all additives, preservatives and food dyes disrupt our intestinal flora and thus affect the immune system. I recommend 'back to basics': use good ingredients, cook your own food, add love to the food. Eat regularly and as much as possible in peace, chew well. These things do a lot for health. With dietary changes, we can definitely affect autoimmunity and the number of antibodies."

Fasting can reduce autoimmunity

Periodic fasting has been much discussed in recent years. Many times, because it can be a way to reduce body fat, but fasting can also help the immune system to get back in balance.

"By letting the body rest from nutrition, avoiding stressful or indigestible foods that trigger inflammation - we give the body the opportunity to begin self-regeneration. This can be supported in various ways, for example, with proteolytic enzymes, with turmeric, black pepper, celery juice or various leafy greens that we know have positive effects in the body.

If you feel that it is difficult to immediately fast for 15 to 16 hours, you can extend the nightly fasting period half an hour per day, so you allow the body to adjust. It can a good idea to skip breakfast because we are such creatures of habit with this meal. We often eat a bread and milk-based breakfast, and it can be difficult for people to think outside of the box. Therefore, it can be easier skipping it. There are also those who skip the last meal of the day."

In Graves', fasting can sometimes be inappropriate, especially when we are very affected by the disease.

"Those who are adrenally fatigued can feel better from eating relatively little and more often. For them, it may not always be a good idea to take a longer break from food. For some people, fasting is not the right thing to do now. They need more frequent meals to function. You can try for yourself and see how it feels in your body."

Dietary changes can be tough

Changing your diet is no minor matter, especially if you eat a lot of the "white toxins" daily. Gunilla knows this and is prepared to offer more support to patients during the transition.

"A challenge when you want to switch to an anti-inflammatory diet and exclude milk and gluten and sugar is to find other alternatives. If you just remove a lot of things from your diet, it feels limited, and then you get a feeling of deprivation. You may need support to find suitable alternatives, not all gluten-free breads are automatically good. There are very many that contain hard processed soy and corn and many additives. You really need to have an awareness when you eat gluten-free but also milk free.

For those of my patients who need more support in their dietary changes, I recommend taking the help of a dietician. When the patient needs continuous support to make lifestyle changes, I refer her to the dietician I work with, Maria Mickelsbacka, or someone else who can give support more regularly."

*

Brenda's story: Changing my diet reduced my eye symptoms

"I was about to undergo surgery to reduce my eye problems when I heard about the possibility of affecting autoimmunity through diet. Even though I had not been interested in living a healthy lifestyle before, I still became curious. I felt that I was at a crossroads and needed to do something to feel better. At first it felt impossible because an anti-inflammatory diet did not resemble how I ate every day. Junk food and soft drinks had to be replaced by a gluten-free diet with lots of vegetables. The most difficult thing was to change behaviour in social situations, it's tough to eat differently than everybody else and say no sometimes when people want to offer me food I do not eat. I also cook more myself, I feel proud to have learned new skills in the kitchen. To be honest, I did not have high hopes for the possibility to influence my eye health, but those I talked to were enthusiastic and convinced me to try. I am glad I took their advice. I never had to have the operation. My double vision is gone, and my eyes are much smaller than before. In addition, I have lost over 15 kilos in weight."

*

Diet to reduce inflammation

Cook the food yourself. You automatically use better ingredients, fewer additives and cook the food more gently.

Carbohydrates with a low glycemic index (GI), which do not give blood sugar spikes. A few tablespoons of apple cider vinegar before the meal or on the salad further lowers the GI of carbohydrates as it causes the gut to be emptied more slowly.

Fatty seafood and fish with a lot of omega-3 reduces inflammation.

Herbs and spices - including turmeric but also many others.

Fruits and berries with strong colours. Blueberries, for example, are packed with anti-inflammatory phytonutrients.

Foods that increase inflammation

Sugar and fast carbs. Keep your blood sugar under control. With high blood sugar, glucose can attach to proteins in the body and cause inflammation.

Trans fats, hiding in processed foods. You should always avoid processed foods, but if it says "trans fats", "partially hydrogenated fat" or "hydrogenated fat" in the list of ingredients, you have an extra reason to not buy them.

Carelessly treated vegetable oils or oils with high levels of omega-6 such as sunflower oil and corn oil. Others are fine – such as oconut oil, avocado oil and olive oil are fine. Use only cold-pressed oils and do not use them for frying, except coconut and avocado. Butter, ghee and lard are also stable while frying in them.

Processed meat. These have additives that affect health negatively and the processing of the meat renders an inflammatory product.

Alcohol. A solvent and can damage the intestinal wall.

Ready-made food. Preferably you buy nothing in the store with an ingredient list. If you still do so, keep in mind that shorter is better.

Gluten, a protein in grains such as wheat and rye. Gluten can, on its own cause leaky gut, create molecular mimicry, increase oxidative stress, and affect the intestinal flora. There are powerful arguments for excluding gluten when you want to cure autoimmunity.

Dairy products. Increased risk of breast cancer, premature death and fractures can result from eating dairy products.

Do not smoke. It is a risk factor for getting Graves' in the first place, including ophthalmopathy, and smoking is highly inflammatory. There is no need to repeat the full list of disadvantages of smoking, you have heard it before. If you smoke, do your health a favour and quit.

Fasting to reduce inflammation

The 2016 Nobel Prize in Medicine went to the Japanese Yoshinori Ohsumi for the discovery of cell breakdown and recycling of its own constituents - called autophagy. Nobel Prize for the discovery of the cell's cleaning service. We can imagine what happens if the cell may not be cleaned at regular intervals. piles of debris ultimately prevent it from functioning effectively. Autophagy is stimulated when the cell experiences a decrease in nutrients, mainly protein. The reduction increases the need to recycle things that are already at hand, and the result is that the cell cleans out waste.

Fasting leads to a reduction in nutrients and induces autophagy. It may sound dramatic to fast, but we all do it every night, when we sleep. There are many variations of fasting, 5:2, 16:8 and fasting mimicking diet are some structured ones. Fasting has been helpful in autoimmune diseases such as rheumatoid arthritis and multiple sclerosis. Patients experienced reduced symptoms and improved quality of life. Another example related to the immune system is that women who fasted for 13 hours each night had a lower risk of relapse of breast cancer. It is not only the longer fasting periods that have an effect, a rule of thumb could be to let the gastrointestinal tract rest during at least 12 hours per day from food.

If you become curious, remember this: when you are in healing for autoimmune disease, be sensitive to what your body can handle in the form of fasting. It is an effort for the body to cope without energy for long periods. Choose one of the easier versions, such as fasting over night for 12 hours to begin with.

Dietary supplements

Above all, you achieve sufficient nutrient status through your diet. That said, supplements can be just that - a supplement to an already nutrient-dense diet. It would be ideal if you could test yourself to see what nutrients you need to replenish, because we are all different. In appendix you will find some suggested tests for nutrient status. Here are some potentially helpful supplements for anyone with Graves':

Vitamin D. For accurate dosing in the individual case, a test it advised. That allows to calculate your personal need for of supplement and the size of the dose. At least 75 nmol/l, though many recommend 100-150 nmol/l, in the blood is linked to the full effect of the vitamin's health benefits. It is not uncommon to need supplements of up to 8,000 IU per day in winter and up to 4,000 IU in summer.

Selenium. Minerals are bound to various molecules to stabilize them in the manufacturing of supplements. Depending on which molecule the mineral is bound to, it is absorbed differently by the intestine. With selenium, 200 mcg of selenomethionine or selenocysteine is your best choice. Selenocysteine has the advantage that it provides extra of the amino acid cysteine, which is necessary for the formation of one of the body's most important own antioxidants, glutathione. Instead of eating supplements, you can eat two Brazil nuts per day, but it does not guarantee that you get 200 mcg as selenium content in nuts vary.

Magnesium. A common nutritional deficiency and causes impaired sleep, tense muscles and problems with metabolism. Magnesium is necessary in over 300 different biochemical reactions in the body. There are different types of magnesium, magnesium oxide is the most common in supplements. Unfortunately, it is not so easily absorbed by the intestine, but is good for constipation. Magnesium bisglycinate is absorbed more easily and is magnesium combined with the amino acid glycine, which is also calming, so this form is usually recommended for sleep and relaxation. Magnesium citrate is also easily absorbed and known to give the positive effects of magnesium.

Iron. Many women are deficient in iron because of low intake of animal foods or loss of the mineral during menstruation. There are several reasons you should keep track of your iron levels: Thyroid peroxidase, which forms T4, depends on iron and your red blood cells, which give you good physical condition, must have the mineral to fulfil their function . Without iron, neither cortisol nor sex hormones will be made, because it is needed when these hormones are built. It is important to use a blood test to find out if you really need extra iron as excess can lead to oxidative stress.

Omega-3. For reduced inflammation, better intestinal flora and building blocks, the brain needs these fatty acids. At least 6 grams per day is associated with better brain health. Find a supplement that is tested to see if it contains flame retardants and heavy metals. If not, avoid it, and avoid any with a report of containing these compounds. Also choose sustainable sources, such as certified fish farming.

B vitamins. Essential for brain health and metabolism. B12 plays a role when T4 is to be activated to T3. B6 and biotin are important in the production of T4. Choose a supplement where the B vitamins are in their methylated, active, form.

Vitamin B	Most active form
B1- Thiamine	Thiamine hydrochloride
B2- Riboflavin	Riboflavin 5'phosphate
B3- Niacin	Nicotinic acid
B5- Pantothenic acid	Calcium D pantothenate
B6- Pyridoxine	Pyridoxal 5'-phosphate
B7- Biotin	D-biotin
B8- Inositol	Myo-inositol
B9- Folate	Methylfolate
B12 – Cobalamin	Methylcobalamin

Glutamine. A deficient product in the body during the disease and an important amino acid for healing the intestines and building muscles and bones and good for brain health.

To increase the levels of glutathione:

Glutathione. Pre-formed glutathione, choose a liposomal variant for best uptake.

Supporters of formation of glutathione. NAC, vitamin C plus several of the above such as B vitamins, vitamin E, selenium, omega-3 and glutamine can help the body form more glutathione.

In addition, if you have recently been diagnosed:

Multivitamin and mineral supplements. Do not skimp when buying multi-vitamin supplements. The cheap ones have nutrients in their cheapest form. This means that you may not absorb the nutrients in the tablet or that your body cannot use it because it is not in an active form. Visit a health food store you trust, they can help you choose a high-quality supplement. If the supplement contains iron, calcium or Q10, take them at least 2 hours apart from your dose of thyroid hormone replacement drugs, as these may interfere with absorption.

Antioxidants. If you have recently been diagnosed with Graves' you can benefit from extra vitamin E, beta carotene, CoQ10 and vitamin C. The minerals selenium, copper, zinc and magnesium are all important in forming the body's own antioxidants. The tyrosine in Q10 can compete with the uptake of hormone replacement therapy so take them separately, at least 2 hours apart.

Myo-inositol, choline and carnitine are all deficient at the time of diagnosis and important for brain health.

Structured diets

There are lots of different diets. All of them have their own promises of what they can accomplish. Here are some diets selected because research has shown that they can help in autoimmune disease or because they have been created by some of the most brilliant clinicians. They have in common that they are anti-inflammatory, heal the gut and balances the intestinal flora.

You are unique and so should your diet be. A tailored diet just for you is ideal. There are ways to get there - elimination diets. Roughly, an elimination diet goes like this: You take a range of foods known to interfere with gastrointestinal health and create inflammation and exclude them for a period. Then reintroduce them, one by one, to see who makes you feel bad, or does not. The result is a diet suitable for you to use when you need to heal. The list of foods to exclude can confuse. Tomato, lemon, and eggs, are they not healthy? Yes, they can be, but they also have properties that sometimes irritate the gut or the immune system, both of which are sensitive because of the disease. Therefore, you who are sensitive to these foods do better without them. When you heal your body, you will tolerate more foods again. The goal is to tolerate as many healthy foods as possible, variety is best. An elimination diet should be done along with other lifestyle measures, such as rest and recovery or physical activity.

Mediterranean diet. The Mediterranean diet is based on how people around the Mediterranean have traditionally eaten. The Mediterranean diet is the diet that is the most researched of all today. The emphasis is on vegetables, fruits, herbs, nuts, beans and whole grains and the meals are based on these. Some dairy products, fish, shellfish, chicken and eggs are also central to the Mediterranean diet. Red meat is rarely eaten. Autoimmune diseases can be improved with the Mediterranean diet and it reduces chronic low-grade inflammation. The high intake of olive oil is highlighted as a reason for the health-promoting effects of autoimmune disease. Following the Mediterranean diet is linked to increased longevity.

Autoimmune Protocol - AIP. An elimination diet based on the paleo diet with a few more excluded foods such as nuts and seeds, and nightshades. The paleo diet says that we should eat the foods we are evolutionarily adapted for and avoid additions we have made in the diet relatively recently, mainly when humans became farmers. AIP has been the subject of several studies and has showed effect in people with autoimmune diseases. Many with autoimmune disease who have tried, testify it improves their health and suppresses autoimmunity. A thorough guide to AIP can be found in "Autoimmune approach: reverse autoimmunity and heal your body" by Sarah Ballantyne.

The Autoimmune Solution. Amy Myers M.D. has written two excellent books about autoimmunity and thyroid: "The autoimmune solution" and "The thyroid connection". Dr Myers has had Graves' herself and has put together guides for prevention and reversal of autoimmune disease. Her program addresses the root causes healing the gut, removing foods that alarm the immune system, lower the toxic burden, heal infections and reduce stress.

CHAPTER 12
BALANCED BRAIN AND NERVOUS SYSTEM

Karin's story: I am grateful for Graves'

Karin Ericsson Back is a freelance singer and you can reach her via the website www.karinericssonback.se. There she writes about life with Graves' and hypothyroidism.

"Graves' disease has permeated many years of my life. I have been tossed around between health care institutions and come across doctors who waved off my symptoms and sent me home with cough medicine. But I have also had care givers that have been worth their weight in gold and given me new dimensions of life. In 2011, I fell ill with Graves' for the first time. Then my body responded quickly to the medication and after two years the drugs were removed, and I was declared healthy. After a car accident in 2017, I fell ill again. In connection with the accident, I received contrast fluid injected into my body before an emergency X-ray examination. Maybe that's why Graves' flared up again? Or was it the stress associated with the accident that triggered it? Anyway, in December 2017, I was diagnosed a second time. I felt so bad - sick, stressed, shivering like a leaf, high heart rate, headache and so sweaty. My thyroid hormone levels were sky high, and I was on sick leave for three months to begin with. Since I work as a freelance singer, I needed to cancel a lot of work. Record recordings, tours, courses - everything I worked hard for, I had to cancel. I cancelled one thing a day, I could not take anymore. I slept, rested, dragged myself out to the mailbox and tried to maintain some kind of routine in everyday life. In April 2018, my endocrinologist told me that the best option for me was have surgery to remove the thyroid gland, something I reluctantly agreed to after reading everything I came across about Graves' and various treatments. An imminent risk was that my voice could be damaged during an operation and I did not want to be part of that nightmare. At the beginning of May, I was admitted for surgery and got the top team of surgeons in one of the university hospitals. In the afternoon, I woke up from the anaesthesia by a surgeon who said that the surgery was cancelled because of one of my vocal cords being paralysed. My right vocal cord had gotten a tear and only half of the thyroid gland had been removed. I fell into a black hole. All the medical staff said that I sounded good and that the operation would surely be resumed the next day. But I felt that something was wrong. When I spoke, it was as if I had an air bubble in my throat that was bouncing. The next morning, I was examined, and it turned out that my right vocal cord was still paralyzed. I was put on a drug to speed up the healing of the vocal cord nerve. The medicine made me dizzy, the blood pressure dropped, and I mostly lay in bed and rested. After a few weeks I got a fever and was hospitalized again. I had thyroiditis, an inflammation that causes the thyroid gland to release stored hormone - one last desperate attempt from it to be productive. An examination showed, however, that my right vocal cord functioned again and then a new surgery was quickly booked. In June 2018, my thyroid was obliterated, and it went without complications. After both surgeries, a long period of rehabilitation of my voice, body and soul followed. I was so scared to use my voice the way I usually do but got wonderful help from a speech therapist, physiotherapist and singing teacher to get it back into shape. However, I was away from the stage for almost a year and a half before I felt ready again. Today I am on a combination of the synthetic T4 and T3 but the road to finding the right dosage was long. And it will most likely need to be changed again as my body changes throughout life. Despite all the tough times Graves' has offered me, I am today grateful for what I have been through. My humility towards life has grown immensely. During my long sick leave, I worked hard to find a more open and positive mindset, which has strengthened me and made me calmer. I plan my life to minimize stress and invest in recovery in connection with intensive work periods. The interest in how my body works has led me to adopt an anti-inflammatory diet, which has helped me in my healing process. Voice yoga is a new discovery that I practice and at the beginning of 2021 I will be a fully trained voice yoga teacher. During the period I could not sing, yoga became a substitute for what I experience when I do concerts - total focus and presence. Because of Graves', I still sometimes have difficulty concentrating, am sensitive to sound and light and am easily frightened. I have a hard time with heat and easily panic when the temperature gets too high. But I am alive and now know that I can manage even if I could not sing. There is so much in life that is valuable."

*

Your brain can change

Contrary to popular belief, the adult brain can change. This applies to the entire brain when new demands are placed on it. Like when we need to repair an injury or learn something new. This is called neuroplasticity. It is never too late to improve brain function, for example, hippocampus can produce new cells throughout our entire lives. Areas that have shrunk, or grown, from stress can be balanced as we recover. When we stimulate it correctly, the limbic system and autonomic nervous system regain their function. An American research group lists three ways to change the amygdala and hippocampus positively:

- Physical activity, read more about this in a later chapter.
- Meditation, preferably with elements of mindfulness.
- Social support and integration.

Meditation to strengthen the brain

Meditation, breathing exercises and yoga can reduce mental illness, change the brain - the same parts that are affected by Graves' - and switch over the nervous system to rest and digest. If you have prejudices against any of the mentioned techniques - drop them and read the following part of the book with an open mind. It would be a shame if you missed that these have the power to change the way your brain and nervous system work.

Meditation can be very relaxing in the moment but is also positive for the brain in the long run. There are an infinite number of types of meditations, some are more well studied than others. Several studies have confirmed that meditation can counteract stress, anxiety, and depression. Objective measures of stress levels, such as blood pressure and the function of the parasympathetic nervous system - heart rate variability (HRV) - improve when we meditate. There are also indications that meditation may be good for the functioning of the immune system.

Studies with patients who have chronic pain or cancer shows that meditation also may improve the quality of life.

Graves' is characterized by changes in the volume of the limbic system. Can meditation be a way to help these areas recover? At present, there is no study that has examined whether specifically patients with Graves' can achieve improvements through meditation or other intervention to reduce stress. But there are studies that show that meditation can change the size of the limbic system. Therefore, it can be an effective strategy to feel better for us with Graves'.

Mindfulness - being here and now

Mindfulness is often included in meditation and is usually said to be one of its most important "active ingredients" to affect our well-being. Mindfulness is about observing thoughts without criticizing and showing compassion for oneself. Things that enter our minds we can try to deal with like clouds passing by in the sky, we look at them with curiosity but do not take them personally. If we can catch negative thought patterns before they bring us into downward spirals of negative emotion, we can gain back some control of our lives. Mindfulness comes from Buddhist philosophy, but has nothing to do with religion. Mindfulness wants to help us see everyday problems in a way that makes us feel more positive emotions. It aims to help us deal with stress and has become popular worldwide. Mindfulness based stress reduction (MBSR) is the most studied type of mindfulness training. People who had never meditated before could use MBSR to influence the size of the hippocampus and amygdala. They also felt less stressed. You do not have to use MBSR to train mindfulness because mindfulness is a feature of many types of meditations.

Besides being examined for its ability to ease mental illness such as depression, mindfulness also has a potential effect on more mundane aspects of our mental well-being: worries, stress, low mood and irritability. Other positive effects of mindfulness may be that you see a doctor less often, your hospital stays will be shorter, you will be more creative, have better memory, better relationships and experience more joy and satisfaction than usual.

Try a mindfulness exercise

Get to know your breathing. If you have never noticed your breathing before, you can try the following exercise where you apply your awareness of breathing. It is also a good relaxation exercise for a stressed mind. Lie down comfortably on your back. Pull up your knees and let your feet rest comfortably on the ground. Then place one hand on your chest and the other over your navel. Breathe quietly through your nose. When lying there breathing, the hand on the chest should be completely still while only the one above the navel moves up and down in step with your breathing. Spend a few minutes getting to know how the breathing feels inside you. Already by observing your breath in this way, you are practicing mindfulness. If you like it, use the observing of your breath in everyday life. It is an excellent way of coming home to your body and calming down. Next, try a more formal mindfulness meditation.

Mindfulness meditation. A common Mindfulness meditation is to observe and follow your breathing. Try this:

- Sit comfortably and close your eyes.

- Pay attention to your breathing and focus on how it feels.
- When you notice that you are thinking of something else, note it without engaging in the thought and start gently concentrating on your breathing again.
- It is important that you bring your attention back to breathing without judging yourself.
- Begin with 3 to 5 minutes, you can build up your practice to 15 to 30 minutes.

Meditation is not about stopping thoughts or having the mind going quiet. It is about discovering where your thoughts are going. Do not be discouraged if the mind wanders, and it seems impossible to concentrate. Each time you find that you lose concentration you bring it back to your object of meditation, in this case the breath.

How much do I need to meditate?

To change the brain, according to research, preferably meditate daily for about half an hour. If you think about all the time you spent being sick and stressed, it's amazing that your body can repair itself just by actively practicing mindfulness and switching to the parasympathetic nervous system for at least half an hour a day. Any time you spend practicing counts, if you cannot do half an hour from the beginning, start with five minutes and build from there. A study of meditation and yoga in combination where the participants received results on brain function showed that the participants practiced for 27 minutes per day on average. Here, participants followed a course in mindfulness based stress reduction (MBSR). If you want to try MBSR, there are free programs to look up online or search for someone who is trained and take a course.

There are many types of meditation. Find one you appreciate and actually will do. If you want to access the calming effect, then choose one where you can feel that you calm down. Try a few different types and note how the effects differ in your body.

How long do I have to wait before I notice any difference?

Quick effects where you feel calm are linked to the individual exercise session. You can enjoy the immediate effects of meditation as soon as you get used to the exercises and start relaxing during them. For more permanent changes, where new nerve cells or nerve connections are required, such as better memory ability or more presence in everyday life, you need to give the exercises up to eight weeks before you feel changes. The brain goes through several stages when it heals itself. It can therefore take six to eight weeks before you notice lasting results from your mental training. If that sounds like a long time, you can take comfort in that you get immediate positive effects from your mental training faster than that. It takes as long for physical exercise to have a deeper effect on brain health such as growing new nerve cells in the hippocampus, at least six weeks, even if you can feel good after a single session.

It is boring and I get jittery when I try to meditate

At first, it is common to feel restless and bored. We are not used to "just sitting". Do not give up, but continue. Probably, we who are more restless during the sessions benefit the most from meditation. Find a guided meditation online or take a course and see if that works better.

Interview with Petra Kalla, Yoga Therapist and Physiotherapist: Strengthening the vagus nerve is well-invested time

Petra Pārvatī Kalla is an C-IAYT yoga therapist and physiotherapist. Her clinical work focuses on mainly mental health, stress related illness and long term pain syndromes. She is interested in guiding people to a more compassionate and informed connection to their body-mind. In her integrative work with Sacred spine yoga therapy, she shares the full palette of yogic practices infused with myofascial release techniques, modern self-compassion based psychology, ancient wisdom teachings of the east as well elements from qigong.

By being interested in the subtle, small and slow – we reach deep within. Listening to the poetic language of our bodies, we honor and heal,
rather than discipline and override our emotional and physiological shifts. The goal is to support people to find the inner will and the tools they need to take care of themselves from the heart.

Petra believes that we should concentrate on the vagus nerve when we want to balance the nervous system and brain after stress.

"We should focus on stimulating the vagus nerve and the parasympathetic nervous system - or the "relaxation response" as this physiological state is also named, because it means that the body is set for recovery and self-healing. The relaxation response, just like the stress response (sympathetic nervous system) affects the entire body and brain at the cellular level.

In research where this response was first mapped, people who meditated were studied while the researchers measured many different things, such as respiratory rate, heart rate, blood pressure, energy consumption, brain waves and more. What they found was, just as we experience it, that the entire body calmed down and required less energy.

An important thing that happens when we relax is that the respiratory rate and the work of the heart are reduced. We get an improved heart rate variability, a kind of coherence between calm even breaths and the heart's pulse variation between inhalation and exhalation. When we breathe 4 to 6 even breaths per minute, our heart rate variability increases. This means that when you breathe in, there is a sympathetic turn-on that makes the heart work a little faster and harder, when you exhale the heart rhythm is calmed via the vagus nerve. We want large peaks and valleys in the pulse variation between inhalation and exhalation. Heart rate variability is related to vagal tone, when they are both high, we know that the body can recover well after stress. High vagal tone and HRV are associated with stress resistance, cardiovascular health and pro-social behaviours. Low vagal tone shows low stress resistance and is linked to disease states such as fatigue, depression, post-traumatic stress disorder, long-term pain and Graves' disease. The important thing, however, is not to have as high a tone as possible, but that the nervous system is flexible and adaptable.

The relaxation response also seems to affect our genes. Studies have shown that immediate changes occur in genes involved in energy metabolism, immune function and insulin secretion."

Many things happen in the body when the vagus is activated because it extends to all the internal organs.

- Increased blood flow to the internal organs
- Decreased metabolism at the cellular level
- Reduced respiratory rate
- Lowered heart rate, lower blood pressure
- Slower brain waves
- Improved sleep
- Improved digestion, secretion of digestive enzymes
- Improved function in our hormone glands
- Normal sex drive.

Petra says that to strengthen the vagus, we should take time to do calm and relaxing activities.

"Some gentle soothing form of movement such as calm yoga, qigong, pai da - self-massage, walking or dancing. Whatever suits you and your body.

Breathing exercises that stimulate the vagus nerve:

Even, slow breathing - Even, calm, simple breaths, 4 to 6 breaths/minute (4 to 6 seconds in/out). Be sure to breathe with the diaphragm, feel the inhalation in the lower chest, abdomen, lumbar spine and pelvis. You do not have to breathe excessively deeply with large volumes of air. Find a comfortable, calm, and quiet breath.

Prolonged expiration - Let your exhalation be longer than the inhalation, about twice as long (for example, breathe in for 4 seconds, out 6 to 8 seconds).

Yoga exercise bhramari (bumblebee) - Inhale calmly and deeply, creating a humming "mmm sound" on the exhale to prolong the exhale. Let the vibration take on a tone that vibrates around the heart in the chest. Singing and voice vibrations are another way to stimulate the vagus nerve.

Each breathing exercise is performed between 5 and 15 minutes.

Guided relaxation training such as progressive relaxation, body scanning, visualization meditations, yoga nidra, self-compassion meditations. The brain gets better at what you practice, so choose meditation with a focus that appeals to you.

Restorative yoga. A meditative and therapeutic form of yoga about relaxing and creating recovery, physically, mentally, and spiritually.

Sing or sound mantras. The vagus nerve lies superficially at the larynx and can be activated by the vibrations when we sing or pronounce the mantra."

On her website, Petra has audio files and videos with exercises: www.sacredspine.se

It is difficult to look stress in the eye

It can be difficult to first take time for these exercise, but once you do it, you notice that the exercises themselves are also challenging.

"The most common obstacle is the stress itself, which is unpleasant to face. First, it is often difficult to make room in the daily schedule, it is so easy to prioritize everything but yourself and your well-being. Stopping and meeting the beating heart, the creeping anxiety and the swirling thoughts are not exactly something we spontaneously long for. It may take some practice relaxing. If you have problems with anxiety and feelings of panic, you may face them when you do relaxation training. What did not want to feel, has a tendency to come to the surface, but this is something positive. By really making room for how we feel, we can develop a new attitude to life."

If you want to overcome the unpleasantness of facing your stress, according to Petra, there are several things to try.

"One of my meditation teachers is a very experienced psychologist, and she has learned to "awaken the inner love in me", so I understand that the inner voice is mine and I can choose how I talk to myself. We often have a judgmental and harsh inner critical voice that is our biggest obstacle. Being aware of how I speak to myself is the foundation for being able to mature emotionally and deal with life's difficulties. Time and time again, capture that voice as it judges and criticizes and practice being kind to yourself instead. Self-compassion is something we can practice and get better at, just like relaxation.

Some other simple and effective things we can do to meet the stress and discomfort is to smile softly at ourselves. The vagus nerve is stimulated by this as it innervates the facial muscles. Putting your hands on your body, massaging or just breathing into them is another way to show emotional compassion for your experience. It is important to release the resistance to the experience. It may not be entirely welcome or exactly what I want but the fact is that it is what is happening. The serenity prayer is so helpful;

"God, grant me the serenity to accept the things I cannot change, courage to change the things I can, and wisdom to know the difference."

In the beginning, it can help to practice with a therapist, someone with experience you trust. For many, it can also be helpful to move the body before doing relaxation, meditation or breathing exercises. Either through a walk, qigong, yoga or dance, whatever suits you. The only way forward on is to keep practicing."

Those who train their vagus nerve get increased knowledge about their body and can reduce their stress, according to Petra.

"It is like learning a new language or playing an instrument, practice gives skill. You learn the poetic language of the body and to play on your inner instrument, your nervous system. This means that over time you become both more stress-resistant and adaptable and less reactive emotionally. Direct effects can be better sleep, less intense and frequent worry and anxiety, reduced muscle tension, better digestion, and increased energy. The effect builds with time. You are required to practice 15 to 30 minutes minimum, almost daily. Make room in your life for some form of regular recovery, something that feels like a gift you give yourself. It is well-invested time, what you get back in the form of increased well-being."

*

Do I need to buy special technology to improve vagus function?

There are equipment and apps for measuring heart rate variability, but you can also learn to pay attention to your body's signals. It can be fun to get confirmation with the help of an app that what you do really helps you get into parasympathetic dominance. However, there are benefits to learning to recognize the signs you are in parasympathetic dominance. Then you have access to that knowledge and can leave the technical stuff behind. Here are some signs that the parasympathetic nervous system is activated:

- Sighing
- Yawning
- Tear flow may increase
- You need to go to the toilet
- The heart rate slows
- You become more sociable
- You feel calm and satisfied
- Muscles relax
- Breath is slower and deeper, low in the abdomen.

Everyday recovery important for vagus

Rest and recovery can be an effective way to break stress here and now, but it is also an effective tool for changing the long-term functioning of our brain and nervous system. Watching TV-series episodes or sitting by your smartphone is not the parasympathetic nervous systems idea of recovering. That is a more active process. It can be about:

- Being physically active
- Meditating
- Eating foods with health benefits
- Listening to relaxing music
- Getting enough sleep
- Being in nature
- Spending time with family and friends.

Social support and integration

A balancing act many of us have to go through is the one between "work-rest-play". When we have a busy schedule, social activities often decrease as a result. These have an important role for health and stress reduction in particular. Differences can be seen in the brain between people with good social support and those without. Positive relationships with friends, family or a partner all count. It is not necessarily the quantity, how many friends and acquaintances we have but quality, do we have someone to turn to with our worries and joys?

Work with social contacts can also give brain the stimulus it needs. A group of older people volunteered to help in preschool and got measurable positive differences in the brain compared to a control group that did not. They spent 15 hours a week for six months helping in preschool. The researchers believe that besides the increased social contact, it was also the meaningful work that contributed to the brain change.

Volunteering also gives a sense of meaning and context. Other ways to take advantage of social contacts are to give and receive touch, seek people with the same hobbies and interests as you, contact friends and family you have not met in a long time. Also nurture the relationships you already have to make them deeper and more meaningful.

There are groups for people with Graves' on Facebook. There you can ask a question or help others answer theirs. It is good to know that you are not alone in suffering from the disease.

CHAPTER 13
RESTORED ADRENAL GLANDS

Interview with Mia Lundin, Nurse Practitioner: Balance the gut and neurotransmitters

Mia Lundin is Nurse Practitioner with specialist training in gynecology and obstetrics and has 29 years of experience working with women's health in the US.

She has founded HerCare, a modern women's clinic with innovative expertise in hormonal health, because she felt that Sweden was far behind in modern, health-promoting and preventive women's health. HerCare wants to change that and offer world class women's health care. You can read more about her at: www.mialundin.com.

Mia Lundin has met many women who are affected by stress and she knows how our bodies react.

"There is a recurring pattern that I have seen through test results in thousands of patients during all my clinical experience. In case of prolonged stress, a period of high cortisol comes first, together with normal or high levels of the neurotransmitters serotonin and GABA. Over time, these decrease. Cortisol no longer has its usual peaks during the day, and serotonin and GABA become low. When serotonin has dropped to a certain level, the feedback system for cortisol does not work. Then we see that ACTH decreases and cortisol decreases. I think it is a defence mechanism that the body has because we have been stressed for too long. Women who are burnt out have very low levels of both GABA, serotonin and cortisol. After prolonged stress, T4 is not converted to T3 but to rT3, the woman then gets a lower T3 value. The sex hormones are also affected by stress, the calming hormone progesterone decreases. Cortisol steals the precursors to the sex hormones. We produce less progesterone and become estrogen dominant. The woman can have heavier periods, at the same time as she experiences an imbalance in her neurotransmitters. Everything is connected."

Many women with thyroid problems come to HerCare and want help to get rid of symptoms and feel better.

"Most people who come to us have hypothyroidism, I've seen a few with active Graves' but it's not as common as Hashimoto's. When a patient has Hashimoto's, we always recommend that they see a nutritionist to reduce intestinal permeability and ensure that they get a healthy gut. Inflammation is reduced and we often see that antibodies drop. We send patients with hyperthyroidism to an endocrinologist because it is an acute condition. Graves' patients can slip into hypothyroidism and then they come to us."

Make a restart to find your way out of stress

When Mia Lundin helps a patient find their way out of stress, it is very much about finding an alternative way of dealing with life.

"The first thing we do is go back to how it all started. We also look at how the woman is feeling, how we can reduce her stress and ask how she ended up here. It is not desirable that she should return to business as usual, because that did not work well for her, but to find a better way to deal with stress and life. Again, we aim to improve gastrointestinal health and increase serotonin. Serotonin and gut are closely linked. If the serotonin decreases, the intestine health worsen and the gut health deteriorates, then serotonin decreases further. Some need talk therapy, others need help with hormonal balance while they recover, maybe they have entered perimenopause because of stress and need progesterone for a while, some have entered menopause and need both estrogen and progesterone. That is functional medicine in a nutshell, giving the body what it needs and removing what should not be there. Actually, it's simple."

Mia Lundin has also seen that women want to try NDT when their symptoms may be due to the fact that they have too much stress in their lives.

"It can be difficult for patients with hypothyroidism to accept that the thyroid gland is not the cause of all their symptoms. NDT is sometimes presented as a "ticket to health". Maybe the last thing a woman needs is more thyroid hormone, her body has converted to rT3 for a reason. She often also has a high resting heart rate, sweating, anxiety and worry - symptoms that she is too stressed and stimulated. Instead, she needs to take it easy and rest. The lower the cortisol, the worse you can tolerate thyroid hormones, the body does not want it then. Instead, we focus on balancing cortisol and neurotransmitters."

Get help if you need it

It can be complex to navigate autoimmunity, stress, and hormone balance. The support of an experienced healthcare professional can help you get ahead.

"Many people come to us for symptoms in perimenopause and menopause and believe that it is the hormones that cause them. In fact, neurotransmitters are out of balance and that is why women feel the way they do. With us she first meets a midwife who charts the symptoms, takes samples, and then the midwife decides if the patient needs to see a gynecologist. She can also get help from a nutritionist with nutrition, gut, and serotonin support through food and supplements. We also have talk therapists, and sometimes the woman needs to meet one of these, sometimes all of them. We also assess whether she needs to see a doctor for other things that are going on, for example thyroid problems."

Easier said than done to relax

Taking time for relaxing sounds easy but can be difficult. Mia Lundin wants to emphasize that the number one thing to achieve recovery is time to rest.

"The most important thing is not to believe that you will feel better because you do high intensity training, instead, you must find peace. Meditate, do yoga, take leisurely walks, look out the window at the birds. Lower the bar. It is difficult for some women, but it is what has to be done. Then improve gut health, give the body the nutrition it needs and make sure it is broken down and absorbed. Be sure to be hormonally balanced in the meantime. Perhaps the body can balance itself, but not if it is in acute crisis. Women who have been burnt out are sensitive, perhaps for the rest of their lives or for a long time. I think the most important thing is to replenish the serotonin. You can do this with tryptophan or 5-hydroxy tryptophan, it works better. You can buy it at for example, hermoodfood.com."

*

Rest for the sake of the adrenal glands

It is not possible to underestimate the importance of stress relief for the adrenal glands to recover. It should be a top priority if you have symptoms that the adrenal glands are not working well. By reducing their need to be productive, they can build up their reserves and the feedback system that has been out of order can function normally again. Things to avoid when you are in any phase of adrenal fatigue:

- Physiological stress, such as fluctuating blood sugar, rapid changes in temperature, inflammation.
- Psychological stress, such as taking on too much to do, worrying, expecting to be perfect.
- Stimulation of the adrenal glands: caffeine, nicotine, alcohol, exercising too hard, sleeping too little.

Use relaxation techniques to recover

Meditation, HRV training, yoga and sleep are perfect for creating a calm environment where the adrenal glands can recover. You can read more about these in the chapter on balancing the nervous system and brain. Those techniques are equally useful for the adrenal glands.

Take control of your blood sugar

When blood sugar drops, the adrenal glands must release cortisol. Cortisol mobilizes glucose stored in the liver, but also stimulates the liver to produce glucose. Avoid fluctuating blood sugar to relieve the adrenal glands:

- Avoid fasting while the adrenal glands are recovering, it places too great demands on them.
- Always eat breakfast, preferably within an hour of getting up.
- Breakfast should be high in protein and fat.
- Eat something every two or three hours and do not wait to get hungry, then your blood sugar is already unstable.
- Choose snacks that contain a low glycemic index. For example: nuts, seeds or root vegetables. Add protein and fat as this slows the absorption of carbohydrates.
- Never eat foods with a high glycemic index without eating protein or fat at the same time.

Learn to sleep again

Sleep is the most recovering thing we can do, it helps the adrenal glands but also all the other systems that are affected by Graves'. Sleep hygiene helps you clear obstacles to good sleep. There are many things you can try, here are some of them:

- Drink all caffeinated beverages before 12 noon, preferably stop completely. Caffeine prevents you from feeling your need to rest, plus it increases cortisol and noradrenaline.

- Sleep restriction. A CBT method that involves limiting the time in bed to sleep better.
- Go to bed at the same time and get up at the same time every day.
- Sleep in a dark and cool room.
- Spend 20 minutes outdoors every day, preferably in the morning.
- Create a routine for going to bed, doing the same things in the same order, every night.
- Stop using screens at least one hour before bedtime.
- Do not eat large meals at least two hours before bedtime, an active digestion can keep you awake. However, if you often wake up at night, you can try to eat something small before going to bed. Preferably a snack with fat and protein, it is absorbed more slowly.
- Physical activity improves sleep, but exercising too hard before going to bed can keep you awake. A walk or some housework in the evening, however, can help you clear your mind and improve sleep.
- Meditation before bedtime increases the sleep hormone melatonin, which helps you sleep well.

Take time off

Do not rush back from sick leave and do not take on more commitments than you can handle. Instead, make fewer. Why are we often in a hurry to return to work after we have been on sick leave? Health and well-being are more important than our work, and we cannot do our best at work if we are not in good shape. Let it take time and ask for more sick leave if you need it. Once we have gone back to work, it can be more difficult to go back on sick leave again. Explain your situation to family and friends. You will do more again, but right now you need all the recovery you can get.

Will Cole, functional medicine expert, reminds us that for the sake of our adrenals, we should learn to say no: "That is still difficult for me. I do not want to disappoint anyone, and there is always more work to do. But managing stress means creating space in your life to recharge, spend time with the people you love and do what you need to do for yourself. Make sure you really make that time. It is as important as anything else you do for your health and maybe more so."

Surviving hormonal swings

Hormonal fluctuations can be stressful and affect us deeply. They can also be increased in amplitude by non-functioning adrenal glands. Books on the subject have titles such as "The Hormone Cure" by Dr. Sara Gottfried, M.D. and "Period Repair Manual" by Lara Briden, ND, to show that we can feel completely upside down when everything is at its worst. These books also discuss the best way to use hormone replacement - bioidentical estrogen and progesterone in premenopause and menopause, which can be positive for the quality of life in hormonal fluctuations. Talk to your doctor to see if hormone replacement may be appropriate for you. There are several reasons we may have hormonal imbalances, and many of them are addressed when you follow the other practical tips in this book. If, for example, you have an underlying inflammation, hormone replacement will mask the problem, but you also need to look at the root causes of your hormonal fluctuations. Studies on quality of life during menopause show that physical activity has an important role, as it can reduce the hot flashes and night sweats that many women find difficult. The bonus is that it is also good for sleep and brain to exercise, more about that in the chapter on movement. Seeking support from others can also be valuable, open up about how you experience these hormonal shifts with other women., we all go through the same phases in life. Phytoestrogens that are found in many plants can stimulate the same receptors as estrogen, although milder, and therefore can form a bridge until your adrenal glands are in balance again. A study showed that women in premenopause who ate more legumes with phytoestrogens had more optimism and a more positive outlook on life. Sources of phytoestrogen:

- Edamame beans and soybeans (choose organically grown and fermented forms of soy but steer clear of highly processed foods with soy)
- Legumes such as beans and lentils
- Ground flax seeds (grind them just before eating so that the fats do not turn rancid)
- Sesame seeds
- Cacao
- Red clover.

Nutrients for the adrenal glands

Replenishing these nutrients can facilitate adrenal gland recovery and provide building blocks for hormone production.

Vitamin C. The adrenal glands are the organs in the body with the largest store of vitamin C. Each time cortisol is secreted, the adrenal glands also send out a dose of the vitamin.

B vitamins. B vitamins are important for the adrenal glands, especially pantothenic acid and biotin and deficiency of these has been linked to poorer function of the adrenal glands.

Minerals. The minerals potassium, zinc, iron, and magnesium are all consumed at a higher rate when cortisol production is high. Magnesium has a special role in giving the adrenal glands a break as it reduces activity in our stress response and thus reduces the need to form cortisol.

Good fats and cholesterol. The steroid adrenal hormones are created from cholesterol, which we get in our diet, or it is made in the liver from fatty acids. Therefore, make sure you get plenty of good fats. Cholesterol is found in eggs, red meat and seafood. Do not worry about getting too much cholesterol. The body reduces its own production when we get cholesterol from our diet

Adjust your carbohydrate intake. Carbohydrates are debated, and the advice points in every direction possible. We all have individual needs for the amount of carbohydrates in our diet. The need depends in part on our metabolic health and how much we move. But genes and epigenetics also come into play. Some convert fats better and others carbohydrates. There are two important reasons you with Graves' may benefit from eating carbohydrates of good quality (that is, non -processed and low GI).

Insulin that is secreted when we eat carbohydrates is needed to convert T4 to T3, which is helpful if you take synthetic T4 as hormone replacement treatment.

People who eat a low-carb diet have higher levels of cortisol. Therefore, when you want to let your adrenal glands rest, you probably need to eat good quality carbohydrates. If you have low energy, see how many carbs and energy you get with your diet.

Women eat too little of nutritious, whole foods. Try to increase the amount of energy and carbohydrates and see how you feel.

Calming herbs and adaptogens. When we lack energy, it is common to reach for herbs and nutrients that stimulate us. Rhodiola and caffeine are two such examples. But if the tank is empty, you have no energy, there is no use in stepping on the gas. Instead you need to give your body a break from doing so much, and rest. Lavender and chamomile support parasympathetic nervous system activation. Valerian, passion flower, hops and lemon balm support GABA signalling, which is our main calming neurotransmitter. Astragalus, ashwagandha, reishi and holy basil are all considered to be calming adaptogens. Adaptogens are herbs that have the ability to help us cope with stress, often through lowering the need of cortisol.

CHAPTER 14
STRONG MUSCLE AND BONE

If there is one miracle cure among lifestyle measures, it is physical activity. Or how about less inflammation, calmer nervous system and balanced brain and strength, cardiovascular fitness and flexibility? Exercise has many more benefits, it is not possible to list them all here. A small study even showed that with physical activity you reduce the risk of relapse in Graves'. The body applies a "use-it-or-lose-it" approach with our physical fitness. In order to stay strong and fit, move and use your muscle and bone. We should therefore make time for physical activity that activates and places demands on the muscles and bones. When we are stronger, we also feel an increased quality of life, the exercise itself can also make us feel better. Everyone who has been physically active probably knows this.

Some would even argue that exercise is the most important habit we can make. Movement gives you a lot of other things in return. A Finnish study showed that physically active people also automatically eat more fruit and vegetables than others. We sleep better and tolerate stress better.

But does exercise also have the potential to help us with some other symptoms, besides muscles and bones, we can get from Graves' disease? Yes, and especially recently, the effects on the brain and nervous system with exercise have been highlighted. Exactly the areas of the brain that are affected by Graves', the limbic system, strengthen with exercise and it can even relieve anxiety and depression. The nervous system also ends up in balance, the parasympathetic - calming part - becomes more dominant when we are physically in shape. For the brain and nervous system, there are several benefits relevant to Graves':

- Release of an important growth factor for brain cells - BDNF and decreased cortisol levels. This stimulates nerve cells in the hippocampus, a part of the limbic system that has shrunk in Graves'.
- Increases the amount of antioxidants in the brain. As we have seen, Graves' patients greatly need antioxidant protection because the levels go down when the disease is active.
- More mitochondria, which leads to the brain working better.
- The calming part of the nervous system becomes more active. The imbalance in the "fight or flight"-response seen in Graves' is decreased and we can feel calmer and more peaceful.
- Muscles can also release mediators that reduce the symptoms of depression.
- Signal mediators in the brain are balanced.
- A single workout can positively affect your mood and if you exercise regularly, you can reduce the risk of depression, sleep problems, memory difficulties, fatigue and much more.

It is never too late to get moving and all movement counts. Then it should only be a matter of beginning to exercise, right? Yes, absolutely, as long as you adapt to how much your body is affected by the disease. The heart, nervous system, muscles and skeleton can be affected in Graves', which requires that the movement is properly adjusted.

IMPORTANT: Rest if your heart is affected

As you know, Graves' has a great impact on the heart. This is also the major reason you need to be careful with movement when you have hyperthyroidism. Be sure to get your doctor's approval to exercise before you begin. Kerstin Brismar, professor of endocrinology, has three points she looks at before approving the patient for exercise:

- "Blood tests of thyroid hormones should be normal.
- Then I examine the patient to see if they feel hot or have palpitations or finger tremors, then they are having a sympathetic surge. Then I usually treat with beta blockers and many feel much better.
- I encourage patients to begin by walking and see how that goes. If the patient gets palpitations or becomes exhausted, that was too much and back off and then gradually increase again."

What do we know about exercise and Graves' specifically?

At the University of Belgrade, a research group has had 52 women, all of whom have achieved normal thyroid hormone levels with the help of treatment, take part in a study on the effects of exercise on function and relapse. One group moved every day for 3 weeks and the control group engaged in other leisure activities. The movement comprised daily walks, strength exercises and stretching. The exercise group received better fitness, lower levels of T4 and higher levels of thyroid hormone binding proteins. They also became less tired, and during a six-month follow-up period, a larger proportion of the training group could end their drug treatment. The difference was 84 percent compared to 18 percent in the physically inactive group. The risk of relapse also decreased, 29 percent compared to 72 percent in the group who did not exercise.

There are several reasons exercise can help Graves':

- Improves your sleep, which is the basis of all recovery and healing.
- Strengthens your limbic system and parasympathetic nervous system, which is good for mental and physical health.
- Helps you take care of free radicals which reduces inflammation.
- Adequate level of physical activity reduces the need for cortisol, which relieves your adrenal glands and balances the immune system.
- And the obvious: it strengthens muscles and bones that have been broken down by the disease.

How should I exercise to strengthen the brain and nervous system?

In his book "The real happy pill", Dr Anders Hansen gives advice on how to exercise for brain health: Exercise at least three times a week so you become short of breath, at about 70 percent of your maximum capacity, 30 to 45 minutes at a time. Continue for at least six weeks. You feel good right after you move, but if you want to feel better around the clock, it takes about six weeks to have an effect. You cannot count on big differences in how you feel the first few weeks. Running - or something just as intense is recommended. Through exercise, you can ease symptoms of ongoing mental illness but also reduce your future risk of it.

Maybe you cannot do intense cardio training right now. Although strength training is less effective in strengthening the brain, it also has a positive effect. Individuals who do not otherwise exercise and begin a strength training program have better brain function than people who continue to live an inactive life.

How should I excersise to strengthen muscles and bones?

Joel Fornander is a physiotherapist and specialist in sports medicine. For over 10 years, he has helped thousands of people improve their performance and recover from injuries. Here he has put together an effective program with workouts you can do at the gym or at home for half an hour. The sessions strengthen muscles and bones.

For most effect from your strength training, train the major muscle groups such as the legs, buttocks and torso. It has the best effects on metabolism, sex hormones and muscle building.

He also emphasizes that we need to train all parts of the body and train alternately to reduce the risk of injury. Also alternate how heavy you train and make sure you have the right technique, so you do not hurt yourself. If you are unsure, you can get help from a physiotherapist to design a training program.

The program is divided into three sessions, two with weights and one without that can be done at home. Spread the training days out during the week to allow recovery between sessions. Short strength training dictionary:

Repetition means the number of times you do an exercise.

Set means the number of rounds of the exercise you do.

Pause for 1 to 2 minutes between each set.

Session 1 - at the gym

Squats, 3 sets and 8 repetitions (that is, you do three rounds with eight repetitions of squats)

Military press, 4 sets with 8 repetitions

Dead lift, 3 sets with 8 repetitions

Bench press, 3 sets with 6 repetitions

Back raises, 2 sets of 10 repetitions

Hanging knee or leg exercises (it is perfectly okay to bend the legs in this exercise), 2 sets of 8 reps

Session 2 - at the gym

Squats, 4 sets with 3 repetitions

Chins (assisted when needed, for example rubber bands) or replace with dumbbell rowing, 4 sets with 6 repetitions

Dead lifts, 4 sets with 3 repetitions

Australian rowing, 3 sets with 8 repetitions

Back raises, 2 sets with 10 repetitions

Hanging knee or leg exercises (it is perfectly okay to bend the legs in the exercise), 2 sets of 8 reps

Use so much weight that you can do all sets and repetitions. The last repetitions should feel heavy without you lacking in technique. When you can do all the repetitions in the set easily, it is time to increase the weight. If you have just been diagnosed with Graves', you may think you are or if you are new to exercise - go slowly. It takes 12 weeks for the body to adjust to all types of exercise. During this period, the goals may be to establish the habit of training and to establish technique and mobility. Then you also have time to listen to your body. Joel Fornander explains:

"Strength training should be challenging to get the best effect. Therefore, if you are a beginner in exercise or affected by the disease, you may need an adjustment period in the first 12 weeks. An adjustment can be more repetitions per set with lower weight. That will be more endurance training, which you then phase into strength training when you lower sets and reps. During the adaptation, you can do 3 sets with 8 to 10 repetitions of all exercises."

Session 3 - at home

Squats or jumps

Push-ups

Sit-ups

Lunges

Bridges or even better chins

Do 3 sets and as many repetitions as you can, of all the exercises.

Be sure to be careful with form and keep your heart rate up. A high number of repetitions give local oxygen deficiency (feels like lactic acid) which gives an increased muscle volume and testosterone release.

Exercising at home can be an excellent alternative, says Joel Fornander.

"If you cannot get to a gym, it is better to train three times at home than nothing at all. According to the research and my experience, two to four sessions per week are good to get the effect of strength training. One workout per week is better than nothing, but you mostly maintain the strength you already have.

To strengthen the bones, focus on training that is weight-bearing and/or gives shocks to the skeleton. Strength training, running and walking before of swimming and cycling. You can also add jumps to your workouts. The shocks activate the bone building."

*

Nutrition for the muscles

Nutrition is a support for the body to help it gain the benefits of the exercise by providing enough building blocks. Here are some important nutrients for muscle function and building:

Protein. If you have read about building muscle, you have probably come across how important protein is, or rather, the amino acids found in protein. Amino acids literally make up our muscles. Make sure you get enough good quality protein. Amino acids that are especially important for muscles are BCAAs - branched chain amino acids. These are leucine, isoleucine and valine. Before and after strength training, eat a snack containing protein with BCAAs and carbohydrates (such as eggs and bananas). It stimulates muscle growth. Foods high in BCAA: chicken, fish, red meat, and eggs. Vegan sources of BCAA can be spirulina, hemp or pumpkin seeds.

Magnesium. Magnesium helps you sleep well, and this is important because our tissues repair and build muscle during the night. It also promotes the muscles to relax and reduces muscle cramps.

Carnitine. Important for energy production and the levels at diagnosis of Graves' are low. Exercise helps the carnitine to be absorbed into the muscles.

Iron. You need enough iron to create red blood cells that carry oxygen to our cells. Without oxygen, not much energy is created in the body. Remember to find out if you really need extra iron as excess can lead to oxidative stress.

Calcium. As the muscles move, they contract and this contraction completely depends on calcium.

Vitamin D. Can help build muscle by balancing our hormone levels, sufficient levels have been shown to improve performance.

Potassium. Helps the muscles maintain the right balance of minerals, which reduces the risk of cramps.

Glutamine. Helps to repair your muscles after exercise. In Graves', the brain has been shown to have reduced glutamine content, and although likely, it is unknown if this also applies to our muscles.

B12. Important for your energy metabolism and for creating red blood cells.

Nutrition for the bones

Your skeleton depends on the right building blocks being available. With the help of a nutritious and varied diet, you lay the foundation for it to get all the nutrition it needs. Important nutrients for building the skeleton:

Vitamin D and calcium are the celebrities for healthy bones. They are important but do not give the full picture of which nutrition is needed for strong bones. Calcium supplements should be in the form of calcium citrate because calcium carbonate requires stomach acid to be broken down. We may have less stomach acid for various reasons, for example, production often decreases after the age of 50.

We get vitamin K2 from the food we eat and our good intestinal bacteria.

Vitamin C and vitamin B6. Needed to form collagen, the body's most common protein and important for structure and durability in tissues - including bones.

Combination of B6, B9 (folic acid) and B12 can help reduce inflammation and strengthen the skeleton.

The minerals magnesium, zinc and phosphorus. Almost half of the amount of mineral in bone is phosphorus.

Omega-3 can reduce inflammation and reduce the activity of the cells that break down bone.

Silica. The mineral has been shown to increase the storage of various minerals such as calcium in the bone tissues and increase the amount of collagen.

Boron. Necessary for the skeleton because it balances our sex hormones, which build up the skeleton, help us absorb magnesium and reduce inflammation.

Phytoestrogens. Estrogen-like compounds - found in plants such as soy, cocoa, chickpeas and red clover. These can mildly stimulate the estrogen receptor, and their intake during menopause is positive for bone mass.

Besides eating well and exercising, you also need to reduce inflammation to slow breakdown and promote build-up of tissues. Acute and chronic low-grade inflammation can adversely affect muscles and bones. We should now take the opportunity to kill the holy cow. Milk has been shown in studies to increase the risk of fractures, rather than prevent them, the researchers suspect that it is because milk causes low-grade inflammation. Yes, you read that right. Milk is not good for bones - in fact, it may increase your risk of breaking them.

When exercise is not working for you

If you previously enjoyed being physically active but cannot be in the same way after the illness, you are not alone. Many women who love to exercise can, after their hyperthyroidism, not do it at the same level. Even those of you who want to get started with exercise for the first time may find that it does not go as you would like. Physical activity is always good, but it may need to be adjusted sometimes. If your favourite way of exercising does not feel good try to find something else you can do. Do not stop completely, it is important to keep the habit of setting aside time for physical activity until you have more strength again. Maybe you can find a new favourite in yoga or strength training if you cannot run or do CrossFit?

Interview with Anna Sparre, dietician and lecturer: Avoid making exercise an additional stress for the body

Anna Sparre runs 4Health where she spreads the message about the truth on how to create health. She runs a health podcast: 4Health med Anna Sparre. There are both Swedish and English episodes. English episodes are generally the b version, at the moment 65b, 93b, 135b, 155b, 159b, 172b, 173b, 192b, 196b, 183b, 202b, 209b, 216b, 218b-221b, 230b, 232b, 248b, 255b-257b.

Anna is a licensed dietician, educated in nutrition at Lund University, in anatomy and physiology at the University of Gävle, and holds a degree in civil engineering from Lund University. She has a past as a professional athlete, as a competitor in the World Cup in kitesurfing, and is also educated in training and exercise, including postural training. Anna's expertise is in nutrition, nutritional physiology, and exercise, and she also works with sleep and stress.

Anna Sparre has helped many clients reduce their stress and believes most people do not understand how it can contribute to making us feel more stressed.

"Many people have an idea from society and the media that more exercise is better. And that the more stressed we are, the more we should train. We have forgotten that we have to listen to our body, this is where it goes wrong with exercise in stress. In the beginning, it can be an outlet for stress, but in the long run it is stressful for the body. Exercise is a form of stress and contributes to the accumulated effect. If we also manage a family, are busy at work and emotional stress - something we worry about - exercise can be the straw that breaks the camel's back."

Anna Sparre usually likens our energy to a savings account for money. The energy savings account should not run out because we need a buffer, but it has done so in case of fatigue.

"Once you have gotten to where you are chronically fatigued, you need to cut back on spending. This often means reducing exercise and especially quitting the monotonous cardio training, such as running, because it is most stressful for the body. I do not mean that you should be sedentary - exercise is good for you, but you need to listen to the body."

Many people can do mobility and strength training even in fatigue, especially shorter sessions. Anna explains what she means by letting the body lead the way:

"Check if the training feels good. If you get exhausted afterwards, it was too much for the body. You may be tired immediately afterwards, but later in the day you should instead feel that you have gained energy from the exercise. Exercise when you are fatigued can go for walks, preferably outdoors in nature, do yoga exercises, strength exercises but keep it short and avoid long cardio sessions. If you need to be still a lot, you can be active by changing position when you rest, for example lying on your belly when reading or writing, or in a yoga position."

No results can be a sign of incorrect exercise choice

If your exercise sessions no longer feel as rewarding, it may be a sign that instead of building your body, it is stressful. Even if we exercise the same way we "always did", it not certain that this particular type of exercise suits our body anymore. Anna Sparre explains how we can notice if the training we do is not right for us.

“The results of exercise can then be absent and instead you get an increased heart rate and the body reacts differently to the training compared to when you were younger. Again, focus on how you feel afterwards. If you get symptoms as if you have the flu or fever and feel tired and crash, it has become far too much.

High levels of stress hormones also make it harder for the body to benefit from exercise.

Some that I have worked with have experienced that even though they exercise a lot, they have a muffin top. Although the primary goal of exercise is not a so-called perfect body, fat storage in the abdomen can indicate high cortisol. When I then ask my clients to skip workouts and just take walks and stretch for a period of time, many come back and have gotten unexpected results. As the woman whose massage therapist asked: " What exercise have you been doing, your muscles are more defined?" the woman replied: “Nothing" Such results can come from a reduction in stress hormones.”

Anna helps her clients to find exercise that makes them feel better and healthier.

“If there is something you like to do - for example dancing, do it. Because even if an activity is stressful, the net effect can still be positive if it brings joy. Then again, avoid monotonous exercise and choose the ones strengthening for the body, raising testosterone and building muscle. Women need it because testosterone decreases with fatigue and age. Do heavier strength training, it does not have to be long sessions, but when at the gym you lift heavy. You can train heavily only with your body weight, through exercises such as push-ups, hand stands and many more. Exercising outdoors is perfect, get dressed and go out and exercise in the garden or a park even when the weather is colder."

Anna concludes by telling us about the importance of sleep for us to tolerate stress, including exercise, better.

"The sleep hormone melatonin is the opposite of cortisol, there is a balance between the two. You may have problems with sleep due to the circadian rhythm being affected. Get out and move in daylight every day, preferably in the morning."

*

Cecilia's story: Exercise did not work for me

"Despite regular training, my physical condition remained the same. I was used to training, and did not recognize my body's responses to exercise. There was no higher gear. When I tried to run intervals for the first time a year after diagnosis, I ended up with hormones completely out of balance. My period came several days early (that has never happened before and not after either) and I felt sick, like I had the flu. Other times, when exercising more intensely than usual, I got sick or had flashing migraines. Instead, after a period of extra recovery, something changed. One day I had decided to ride the bike to my family doctor. I had to take samples of my thyroid hormones. Through the forest there was a shortcut to the health centre that I had not tried before and off I went. Once in the forest, I had to drag the bike over roots and rocks, cycle up steep slopes, and still I arrived late and sweaty to my doctor's appointment. I left the bike outside the reception and picked it up with the car later in the evening. Normally, such an effort would have backfired. But this time it was different. My body responded to the effort, and I got in better shape. I am convinced that my extra recovery led me to increase my physical capacity. I have finally learned that training is not primarily about performance. It is a way to feel good and strengthen my health. If I had been able to give myself advice when I was fruitlessly exercise in the beginning, it would be to do something else. Find something that the body responds to, no matter how small. And spend more time in recovery."

*

I feel exhausted - should I exercise?

Fatigue in Graves' has several potential causes. What they all have in common is that they limit the body's opportunities to have energy for movement and gain the benefits of exercise. Check with your doctor that he or she gives you approval to exercise. Then your most important tool is to listen to the body and work on the other imbalances mentioned in the book. Adrenal glands that do not function properly, inflammation that breaks down the body or an out-of-balance nervous system may need to be addressed before you feel that exercise is rewarding for you. A basic rule is that exercise should provide energy, not drain you. Also keep track of how the training makes you feel not only the same day but also the next day. Find something you enjoy and feel good about. Everything counts, remember that.

My muscles burn already at light exertion and burn even the next day?

When we are physically active, the demands on the muscles to generate energy increase. Energy formation can take place with oxygen, or without. When we generate energy without oxygen, it is a quick way to get fuel, but it comes at a price: lactic acid. When too much lactic acid accumulates, the muscles become tired and we experience a burning feeling. The mitochondria are the place where energy formation with oxygen takes place. If the mitochondria are affected, you may need to generate more energy without oxygen during physical activity - which increases the risk of lactic acid. In normal cases, this happens when we sprint or do other high-intensity training, but it can happen with low effort. Give the body time to recover, proper nutrition and rest. For now, you can perform exercises that do not trigger lactic acid accumulation. Heavier strength training is one such example. Try to do fewer repetitions of strength exercises, but with higher weights. Women with fibromyalgia, where accumulation of lactic acid is part of the disease, have been helped by heavy weight training with fewer repetitions. Cardio training more easily triggers lactic acid accumulation, but try walking and if you want to run, you can see how much you can tolerate. Start by running for a few minutes and see how you feel.

Begin exercising

You have the motivation and ambition to exercise but do not know how to get started. Here are some tips:

- Plan your training and book an appointment with yourself.

- See yourself as a person who exercises regularly. How does such a person behave? Try to imitate. Identifying with your habit can increase the chances that it will stay.
- Try to train the first thing you do in the morning, it can increase the chance that it will happen. Take out your workout clothes in the evening. If you need to before the workout, eat something small that does not weigh you down.
- Plan in advance what you will do at each session. Do not start thinking about it once you have time for exercise.
- No one wants to train each time a workout is scheduled. Tell yourself to try it for 10 minutes and then decide if you do the whole workout or cancel it.
- Contrary to many people's beliefs, inner motivation is crucial to establish a training habit. Reasons such as health and well-being are more motivating in the long run than looking good. Think about your inner reasons for exercising.
- Do not underestimate sneaking in exercise. Walk or bike where you are going, walk up the stairs, stand up to stretch at your desk and use a standing desk.
- Find exercise you like and makes you feel good, that increases chances that you will do it.
- Exercise so you become sweaty for half an hour a day and mix cardio with strength training. For example, running on one day and a workout with free weights the other.
- Are you more motivated if you train with others? Then make sure someone is waiting for you by the running track or at the gym.
- Exercising at home is an excellent option if you do not want to go to the gym or if time is short. There is plenty of inspiration online for exercising at home without equipment.

CHAPTER 15
ACCEPTING FRAME OF MIND

Lena's story: Life becomes what I make it

"When I first learned that I had Graves' disease and endocrine ophthalmopathy, it felt like the world ended. I could not understand how it was possible that I suffered from autoimmune disease, that my body attacked itself.

During my first period of illness I had powerful fears and anxiety about what life would now be like. I tried to read as much as I could to understand what had happened and how I could help myself heal. I made several radical changes in my lifestyle but saw small results.

It took me over a year to realize that life would never be the same. That much of what I had previously taken for granted was no longer possible. Today I have realized that I have two choices. Either I continue to strive for the impossible or I make the best of the situation I am in right now. And I have chosen the latter.

Mindfulness is my primary tool for making the most of every day, and I have realized that there is often an opportunity to rest and experience beauty in being present. Although my life is so different compared to before the disease, today I feel a gratitude for what the disease taught me and for the life I have today.

It is a tough and challenging journey to realize that life will never be the same. That what I previously took for granted is no longer possible. But I have realized that I have a choice in all this. That I can make the best of the situation, as it is. Live by the values that are most important to me. Savour the moments of joy of life I get, even during the periods when they are rare.

This is my salvation in this new life situation. To enjoy the moments with my children, listening to the birdsong and really experience the wonderful scents of the seasons. Living consciously and continuing to practise being here and now every day is the only way for me to live my life the way I want to live it. And suddenly the disease becomes easier to bear. For the disease is not what defines me. What I make of my moments is who I am."

*

Part of being human is experiencing mental or physical illness. It is inevitable, but we can practise dealing with ill health in a way that reduces our suffering and increases quality of life. It can be frustrating to live with symptoms of an illness that do not lift whatever we do. We do not control everything that happens in our lives and cannot, for example, intentionally make the immune system stop attacking our own body. When we have done everything right, and sometimes we must not see it as a sign that we are failing if we are still not feeling well. Health is not something we perform, it is far more complex. Countless factors must be taken into account, many of which we cannot influence.

If you have Graves' ophthalmopathy or have been treated with radioiodine, you have a greater risk of living with a reduced quality of life than the rest of us. Your need to find constructive ways to deal with illness can therefore be even greater.

When Lady Gaga discussed her approach to her symptoms of mental illness and fibromyalgia - radical acceptance - she opened up the discussion on any suffering from disease that we wish we did not have to battle. Oprah summed up radical acceptance as: "Wanting something to be what it isn't," and realising that "it doesn't change until you first accept it for what it is." Lady Gaga's own way of framing her difficulties in experiencing mental health issues was: "I have radically accepted that I will put my shame in a box all the way over there, and make it very small, and say to myself, I have mental health issues. I take a lot of medication to stay on board and I am a survivor. I am living and I am thriving and I am strong and I am going to take all my life experiences and I am going to share them with the world and make it a better place". If you want to watch their entire discussion, do a search online for "Oprah's 2020 Vision Tour Visionaries: Lady Gaga interview".

Quality of life in chronic disease

Illness that lasts for a long time, even becomes chronic, can lead to a reduced quality of life. This is not to say that everyone with chronic disease has their quality of life reduced. In the introduction, we discussed that it is entirely possible to be classified as ill but still feel relatively well. What determines whether a person experiences a reduced quality of life as a result of illness or not? Psychological factors such as your own perception of the disease, coping strategies (how you handle it), self-efficacy (how well you feel that you are dealing with the given situation), psychological flexibility (being able to shift attention and perspective instead of getting caught up in certain thoughts and action habits) as well as the ability to regulate emotions have been shown to be important in explaining the differences in perceived quality of life. A review of randomized and controlled trials with over 1,200 participants examined the effects of different techniques aimed at increasing mindfulness and acceptance as a way of dealing with chronic pain. The researchers could see that the effects can vary between individuals, but that these can be excellent alternatives in chronic disease. Here you are introduced to two techniques to increase mindfulness and acceptance.

Practicing acceptance

The founders of Acceptance and commitment therapy (ACT) write in their book "A liberated mind - the essential guide to ACT" that we like to put labels and diagnoses on human suffering when the cause of the suffering is obvious - it is difficult to be human. A common equation is that Suffering = Pain x Resistance to the pain. By reducing the resistance, we can reduce the suffering. We can have both unpleasant and pleasant thoughts, that is normal. It is when we let thoughts and feelings completely dictate us, we get lost. The most important thing we can do is accept instead of avoiding emotions. Acceptance promotes, according to the authors, psychological flexibility and compassion. We observe the mind and embrace the moment. In summary, it can be said that ACT puts together conscious presence, values and actions to provide psychological flexibility.

In chronic conditions, many believe that ACT is a useful therapy to increase quality of life. Negative ideas about the disease can be realistic. Therefore, ACT focuses on promoting the behaviours the person values while accepting the negative ideas. Avoiding thoughts about shame and fear has been suggested to be the reason we do not follow the advice about treatment we receive from healthcare. Therefore, ACT can help both manage the disease psychologically and take care of the physical aspects.

"I think" - An ACT exercise

Think of a difficult thought with the form "I am X". It can be "I am unsuccessful" or "I am worthless". If you can, use one that often comes up for you. Concentrate on that thought and believe in it all you can for ten seconds.

Now put "I am thinking" in front of the other words. Now the sentence is: "I am thinking that I am worthless ". What happens inside you then?

Add a few more words: "I notice that I am thinking…". Then what you say to yourself is: "I notice that I am thinking that I am worthless". Did it make any difference inside of you? The purpose of the exercise is for you to distance yourself from your thoughts, to not believe in them blindly.

Here are some more ways you can practise accepting your situation:

- Be mindful of when you are resisting or fighting reality. It is common to wish that symptoms should disappear, that they are unfair or just don't fit your expectations for your life.
- Some things cannot be changed. Your job is to identify what you can change and focus on that.
- Use your body to facilitate acceptance. Notice where you are tense and allow muscles to relax.
- Allow negative feelings to surface. Although no feelings are negative, they all have a message for us, we often experience anger or grief as less pleasant. Accepting may mean that such feelings appear in your mind. Try not to bury them, but to allow them to be there without judgment.
- Show to yourself that you accept your situation. Do this by engaging in a behaviour that you would do if you mastered

acceptance, even when you feel that you do not. Acting as is can strengthen your identity as someone who is accepting.

Compassion-focused therapy

Compassion is a sensitivity to suffering of self and others with a deep commitment to relieve it"

Dalai Lama

Compassion comes from Latin and Greek where it means to go through, or experience. The concept is often associated with Buddhist philosophy, but it is an important element in all the major world religions. It can be unusual for us to aim compassion towards ourselves, that is not something we normally practice in the western culture. Self-compassion according to researchers has three parts:

- Caring for yourself. Instead of being self-critical, you can be a support to yourself, offer a comforting word or give yourself a break when you need it.
- Affinity. Not to let suffering become something that shields you from the environment but brings you closer because suffering is something all people go through.
- Mindfulness. You are present without being completely consumed with your suffering.

Exercising compassion and powerful connections with other people can be a great way to strengthen the vagus nerve. The research that confirmed this used a meditation called loving-kindness (the meditation is available as an exercise below). In it, you focus on creating positive feelings for yourself and others. A different study found that a group had to reflect on their positive social relationships and how to strengthen them, also received increased vagal tone.

Compassion can be described as a mental state that is facilitated by developing various qualities and skills:

- Motivation, to increase your well-being and reduce suffering.
- Sensitivity, listening to your actual needs.
- Sympathy, share joy and sorrow with yourself and others.
- Empathy, you can understand the feelings and suffering of others but are not "infected" to the same extent by the person's experience.
- Tolerance of discomfort, enduring that life offers situations you experience as negative.
- Non-judgmental, not putting values in or judging what you feel, think and experience.

Also practice:

- Attention, to consciously direct your focus.
- Reflection, use your ability to reflect helpfully.
- Acting, to behave in a way that reduces your own and others' suffering.
- Body awareness, the body is a gateway to emotions and by activating the parasympathetic nervous system, compassion is facilitated.
- Visualize, use sight or other senses to experience compassion.
- Emotional regulation, warm and friendly feelings for yourself and others.

Treat yourself with kindness - An exercise in compassion

Treating ourselves with kindness can be a way to feel calmer and more satisfied with life. But how kindly do you talk to yourself?

Do you usually tell yourself that you should feel differently than you do?

Do you look down on yourself for how you think?

Do you usually judge your thoughts as abnormal or bad?

Do you view your emotional reactions as irrational and wrong?

Do you evaluate your thoughts and feelings as either bad or good?

If yes, you can benefit from practicing loving-kindness towards yourself.

Try a loving-kindness meditation

Begin by noticing your breathing.

Try to aim compassion towards yourself. If it helps, think of a person you have warm feelings for. Imagine looking into their eyes and seeing their love for you. See yourself through their eyes and feel love and compassion for yourself. You can also think of yourself as a child and direct the love to the child within you.

Try to say within yourself: "May I live with ease, be happy and free from suffering."

Note that it should not be a focus on external qualities (for example, that you have a nice car) or self-esteem (I perform so well). It is about developing a non-judgmental goodwill and compassion where everything is allowed, beautiful and less beautiful qualities.

Continue if you want by directing the same compassion to a person you have warm feelings for, someone you are neutral towards like someone you meet on the street and finally a person you are having a conflict with. Finish by taking 10 conscious breaths. Start by practicing for 5 minutes and preferably increase up to 15 minutes.

Thinking positively is not necessary

Do you place demands on yourself to think positively about your illness but fail? And therefore, you accuse yourself even more, when now you cannot even visualize how you will regain health? Remember that positive thinking can manifest itself in the small things. Picking up and reading this book, for example. It shows that you hope and believe that there is something to do in your situation. That might not mean that you will be declared healthy and get rid of all symptoms. An acceptance of the current situation can be as valuable in helping you enjoy life more. Acceptance is not about giving up and surrendering. Instead, it is about doing what is in your power to feel better and then accepting any remaining challenges you have. Let acceptance inspire you to take command of your health and take care of your body in the best way.

"Nothing will work for you if you do not do it"
Maya Angelou

My story: From well to vital

I sometimes wonder if I can claim to be 100 percent recovered from the disease or not. It has taken me five and a half years to get to where I am today in the pursuit of more vitality. Do I have the energy to do everything I want? No - but how many do? Can I do everything Ineed to keep my daily life and family happy? Yes, I can. To also take into account is that since my diagnosis I have become five years older, with two small children. How much energy would I have had even without the disease? Another question is if I even want to be the woman I was before the disease. She was too stressed out and although she was aware of what is important in life, she did not prioritize it. More than a full-time job, a large house in need of renovation and unnecessary consumption drained valuable life force. Life with new priorities looks different. We have moved and have more family time. The disease has made me do less and be more, I feel that other parts of life are richer. So no, I do not want to be her. I do not want to be without the disease either, on the contrary, I am grateful for it. I have met amazing people and I am living a life closer to my values, thanks to it.

What I can notice, is that once every now and then, I suddenly get additional energy I did not feel I had before. Recently, I have had another breakthrough in my energy levels and my physical capacity, five and a half years after diagnosis. It came after a period focusing on relaxation and lots of time for my family. My firm belief is that rest comes first for us with Graves'.

PART FOUR – APPENDIX

APPENDIX A - USEFUL LAB TESTS

After applying lifestyle changes, symptoms often improve and there is less need for lab testing. Implement the root causes of health and stay on course for a few months, if you still see lingering symptoms - this is when lab tests may come in handy. Sometimes though, they may be useful right away and always follow the advice from your health care practitioner on what tests to take. Tests may be available as home tests or blood tests, for which you need the help of a health care provider to take. Online companies offer services where you can order a blood test and have it taken at your health centre.

Thyroid

With thyroid testing, you want to make sure not only to test TSH. As that is only one piece of the puzzle. Your free T4 (fT4), free T3 (fT3), reverse T3 (rT3) and thyroid antibodies are also important.

TSH. The hormone that the pituitary uses to tell the thyroid to make more hormone. In active Graves' this may be so low it cannot be measured. Ideally is should be in lower range. In many countries, levels of up to 4 mIU/ml are accepted which by many is considered far from optimal. A research study suggests that between 0.5 mIU/mL and 2.50 mIU/mL is better for patients wellbeing. Amy Myers writes in her book "The thyroid connection" that she wants to see levels of between 1.0 mIU/mL and 2.0 mIU/mL for her patients.

T4 and T3. T4 is the precursor of the active hormone T3. Normally in hormone replacement, the ratio of T4 to T3 is lower than for people running on their own thyroid hormones. These tests will let you know if you have enough hormone to cover your body's needs. If they are high, this indicates hyperthyroidism and if they are low, this indicates hypothyroidism.

rT3. The level of rT3 will indicate at what rate the body wants to protect you from thyroid hormone. This can happen when we are under stress or if you have a low energy intake. If the other thyroid tests are normal, but you have hypothyroid symptoms, a high rT3 value may give clues as to why that is.

Thyroid antibodies. In Graves', the most important antibody is TRAb. This stimulates the TSH-receptor in the thyroid and makes it produce excessive amounts of hormone. Many with Graves' also have high levels of TPO and TG antibodies. That indicated that you are at risk of developing Hashimotos' thyroiditis, the most common type of hypothyroidism, in the future. Make sure to test your levels of thyroid hormones and antibodies regularly.

Nutritional deficiency lab tests potentially useful in Graves'

Aim for a combined test that measures several markers at the same time. Usually this includes both vitamins and minerals but also a blood count test. The number and volume of your blood cells will give information on your nutritional status.

Vitamin D - a common deficiency and many have levels in suboptimal ranges.

Hemoglobin and ferritin - show the need of iron supplementation.

Selenium - this mineral is crucial for thyroid function, and often our food does not contain the amounts we need.

Vitamin A, zinc and magnesium are all important for thyroid function.

Methylation panel -this will allow testing for the need of supplementing with B-vitamins and the level of inflammation. A methylation panel might imply the need for further lifestyle changes and includes markers of:

- Methionine
- Cysteine
- S-adenosylmethionine (SAM)
- S-adenosylhomocysteine (SAH)
- Homocysteine
- Cystathionine
- Ratio of SAM to SAH

Organic Acids test - While the methylation panel is usually a blood test, the organic acids test is a home test based on urine. It will give you some information from a methylation panel and status of antioxidants depleted in Graves':

- Functional vitamin and mineral status
- Amino acid insufficiencies like carnitine and NAC
- Oxidative damage and antioxidant need
- Phase I & Phase II detoxification capacity
- Functional B-complex vitamin need

- Neurotransmitter metabolites
- Mitochondrial energy production
- Methylation sufficiency
- Lipoic acid and CoQ10 status
- Markers for bacterial and yeast overgrowth

Even though inflammation marker homocysteine is not included, the level may be interpreted from the levels of B-vitamins. Sufficient levels of B-vitamin metabolites will help you assume that homocystine is not accumulated. A skilled practitioner can help you get a lot of information from an organic acids test not written in the test result. Not all tests include the above mentioned markers, check before ordering the test.

Central and parasympathetic nervous system functionality

HRV testing will allow you to assess whether your parasympathetic nervous system has been weakened by the disease. Heart Math or a similar device will guide your training. If you do not want to buy the gear, visit a practitioner skilled in HRV testing.

Neurofeedback. Although not discussed in this book, neurofeedback can be helpful in allowing your brain getting back to a calmer, more mindful state. On the one hand, there are home devices for this purpose, although it is not sure how reliable these are. Neurofeedback with a practitioner, on the other hand, can be expensive. Rest assured that your dedication to meditation or a similar brain training practice will improve the state of your brain waves, neurofeedback assessments or not.

Blood sugar

Fasting blood glucose, fasting insulin and Hemoglobin A1c (HBA1c) will give you an idea of the need for implementing measures for blood sugar control. If you find an imbalance, take it seriously as this might contribute to most chronic diseases.

Gut imbalances

Leaky gut is implied when you are suffering from autoimmune disease. This test is therefore often not necessary and what you should do is work on the root causes of health. The test is a urine test where you drink a combination of two sugars (mannitol and lactulose). One is small enough to pass a healthy intestinal lining and the other normally cannot pass because it is too large. However, in leaky gut the intestines become more permeable and larger molecules may pass. A high ratio of the large sugar molecule in urine means that the gut is leaky.

Gluten intolerance or celiac disease. Some say that anyone with Graves' should be tested for gluten intolerance since they so commonly appear together. If you want to test for gluten intolerance, please remember that you cannot exclude gluten before the test since this will prevent antibodies from appearing on the lab result. Also, you do not have to be gluten intolerant to benefit from a gluten-free diet since it can affect inflammation and gut health in all of us. This should therefore not be used as a test to see if you can eat gluten or not. If you suspect that your body does not rhyme with gluten, do an elimination of any foods containing it and see how you feel. Let your body guide you.

SIBO. Dysbiosis in the gut can be a cause of many persisting symptoms. Finding out the presence of any uninvited pathogens in your gut and escorting them out, can be a way of healing. The test involves drinking lactulose and then wait for to see if it is metabolized into any of the gases significant for upper intestine infection. All pathogens require their own specific protocol to be removed from the gut, and you are advised to work with someone skilled in balancing gut flora to get the best results.

Hormonal imbalances

Cortisol imbalances are often at the root of hormonal imbalances, also for sex hormones.

Saliva testing of cortisol. A 24-hour saliva test can be done at home. The result shows the diurnal rhythm of cortisol and hormone levels. Therefore, you will learn not only if your adrenals secrete enough of the hormone but also if they do it at the right time of day. Cortisol levels are highly variable and influenced by what is going on during the particular day of the test. It indicates adrenal functioning.

Dried Urine Testing. Allows for testing levels of sex hormones, cortisol and selected organic acids. This can be done as a home test, but the interpretation is complex since so much data is provided and it is recommended to be guided by a skilled professional.

Chronic infections

As you know, several pathogens can cause a chronic infection and in the long run autoimmune disease. Here are some of the most common tests to find chronic infections:

Epstein Barr Virus. Test for current and chronic infection.

Helicobacter Pylori. These bacteria are perhaps most known for causing stomach ulcers, but is common in any gut imbalance and autoimmune disease. It is a part of our normal flora, but in excess it will cause problems. If you have symptoms of indigestion difficult to resolve, you may have an infection of H. Pylori.

Lyme disease. This infection is growing more and more common because of climate changes. An infection can be limited to the skin, but Lyme disease can affect the nervous system and Borrelia Burgdorferi, the bacteria causing lyme disease, can become dormant and the infection chronic. Testing is controversial and can be complex.

What about genetic testing?

Genetic testing, mainly of so called single nucleotide polymorphisms (SNPs), is popular to learn individual risk factors of accruing certain diseases. While there are a few DNA markers of serious diseases, the SNPs are natural variants of DNA that can influence health. But knowing your DNA does not tell the entire story. As you learned before in this book - genes load the gun, but environment pulls the trigger. What that means in practice is that someone with a poor set of genes, but a healthy lifestyle may never suffer the consequences of their so called "bad genes". Many functional medicine practitioners also point out that they never "treat SNPs" - meaning that they will not base supplement or lifestyle recommendations on DNA testing. Instead, what they do is find out the actual levels of B-vitamins or detox pathway functioning. Then they will suggest a protocol for correcting any imbalances. Other practitioners use DNA testing to probe for potential weak spots but still rely on functional testing to guide the protocol they make for you.

However, it is human to be curious of your DNA. And if you find out you metabolize stress hormones more slowly or have in inherited increased risk of oxidative stress, it may motivate you to implement lifestyle changes. In that case, go for the DNA testing - as long as you remember that there is no use in treating SNPs.

APPENDIX B – SUPPLEMENTS IN GRAVES' DISEASE

WHEN TO USE	DOSE	NOTES
THE BASIC PACKAGE		
Vitamin D	2000 – 5000 IE/day	Take a blood sample to know your exact dose
Selenium	200 mcg/day	Vital for reducing inflammation and improving thyroid function
Magnesium	200 mg/day or more if needed	Choose magnesiumbisglycinate or magnesiumcitrate
Iron	50 to 100 mg/day elemental iron. Use testing to	Supplement only if deficient as too much iron causes oxidative

	monitor ferritin levels	stress. Can cause constipation and dark, hard stools.
B-vitamins	Good B-vitamin complex with methylated forms	Can restore cortisol levels, energy production and conversion of T4.
Glutamine	6-18 g/day	Heals leaky gut and this amino acid is deficient in patients with Graves'
Glutathione	400 mg/dag	Antioxidant that does many jobs for thyroid health
N-Acetyl-L-Cysteine (NAC)	1800 mg/day	Supports glutathione production
Vitamin C	750 mg/day	Supports glutathione production, hormonal

		balance and adrenal health
CoQ10	100 to 400 mg/day	Highes doses when thyroid levels are high. Some may feel stimulated by CoQ10
Omega-3	1000 to 4000 fish oil mg/day	Choose a clean source that is considerate of the environment
BASIC PACKAGE EXTRAS FOR NEWLY DIAGNOSED		
Multivitamin and mineral supplement	Good complex of high quality	Nutrient deficiencies right after diagnosis often include many different nutrients
Vitamin E	50 to 400 mg/day from a source with all types of	Protects lipids from oxidative stress

	tocopherols and tocotrienols	
Beta carotene or Vitamin A	7500 µg beta carotene which is the precursor of Vitamin A or Vitamin A 2000 IU	Protetcs from oxidative stress. Some of us do not convert beta carotene well to Vitamin A. It may therefore be best to choose Vitamin A.
Zinc	Up to 50 mg/day	Supports the production of endogenous antioxidants
Copper	2 mg per day	Supports the production of endogenous antioxidants
Myo-inositol	2 g/day once or twice per day	Supports adrenal and brain health

Choline	250 mg/day	Important for brain health
Carnitine or Acetyl-L-carnitine	500 mg/day	Cartnitine converts into Acetyl-l-carnitine. Acetyl-l-carnitine is the form primarily used in the brain but can be stimulating for some.
BRAIN SUPPORT		
Polyphenols	Found in: Cloves and other herbs like peppermint, oregano. Cocoa and coffee, Berries. Non-berry fruits. Beans. Nuts. Vegetables. Soy.	If you are newly diagnosed of sensitive – skip coffee, chocolate and tea. There are so many other ways to get your polyphenols.

	Black and Green tea.	
Omega-3	1000 to 4000 fish oil mg/day	Choose a clean source that is considerate of the environment
ALA	300 to 600 mg/day	Powerful antioxidant
Carnitine or Acetyl-L-carnitine	500 mg/day	Cartnitine converts into Acetyl-l-carnitine. Acetyl-l-carnitine is the form primarily used in the brain but can be stimulating for some.
CoQ10	100 to 400 mg/day	Highes doses when thyroid levels are high. Some may feel

		stimulated by CoQ10
Cholesterol	300 mg/day	Found in foods such as eggs. meat and avocado.
B-complex	Choose one with high quality and methylated forms	Supports neurotransmitter production.
Phosfatidylserine	200 to 400 mg/day	Improves mental focus, memory, and mood.
ADRENAL SUPPORT		
B-complex	Choose one with high quality and methylated forms	Supports production of cortisol
Vitamin C	1000 mg/day	Adrenals are the organs with the

		highest store of Vitamin C
Calming adaptogen complex	High quality that promotes sleep and relaxation	Avoid stimulating adaptogens
Lavender and chamomile	As tea or tincture	Promotes activation of parasympathetic nervous system
Valerian, hops, lemon balm and passion flower	As tea, supplement or tincture	Activates calming brain cell signalling
MUSCLE SUPPORT		
Vitamin D	2000 – 5000 IE/day	Take a blood sample to know your exact dose
Protein	At least 0,8 g/kg bodyweight per day	Protein literary make up muscle and other supporting tissue

Magnesium	200 mg/day or more if needed	Choose magnesiumbisglycinate or magnesiumcitrate
Iron	50 to 100 mg/day elemental iron. Use testing to monitor ferritin levels	Supplement only if deficient as too much iron causes oxidative stress. Can cause constipation and dark, hard stools.
Carnitine or Acetyl-L-carnitine	500 mg/day	Cartnitine converts into Acetyl-l-carnitine. Acetyl-l-carnitine is the form primarily used in the brain but can be stimulating for some.
Calcium	1000 mg/day	Choose calcium citrate for higher bioavailability
Potassium		

Glutamine	5 grams 1 to 4 times/day	Begin with the lower dose and increase from there
BONE SUPPORT		
Calcium	1000 mg/day	Choose calcium citrate for higher bioavailability
Vitamin K		Also feed your healthy bacteria as these can make vitamin K calc
Vitamin C	1000 mg/day	Hels form collagen, important for bone
Magnesium	200 mg/day or more if needed	Choose magnesiumbisglycinate or magnesiumcitrate
Zinc	Up to 50 mg/day	Supports the production of

		endogenous antioxidants
Phosphorous	700 mg/day	Fish, meat and eggs are good sources.
Omega-3	1000 to 4000 fish oil mg/day	Choose a clean source that is considerate of the environment
Silica	700 mg/day	Supports muscle and bone
Boron	3 mg/day	Hormone balance, important for strong bones, is dependent on boron
Phytoestrogens	30 to 150 mg/day	Extract from soy, red clover or flax seeds.

APPENDIX C - DIGGING DEEPER. WHAT TO DO WHEN YOU ARE NOT FEELING BETTER

When you have done everything in your power but are still not getting better, it is all too easy to lose hope. With no improvement in sight, we might give up on lifestyle changes and feel like it was all a waste of time and energy. If only everyone had a few simple tweaks to make and Voila, we were beaming with health and energy. Thyroid autoimmune disease is complex, and you have learned in this book that it can have a domino effect on your health.

We who have had Graves' not only risk it reappearing and cause symptoms to return, but we are at greater risk of other autoimmune diseases, commonly Hashimoto's. Besides that, we may have an increased risk of heart disease, mental illness, chronic infections, and osteoporosis. These are associated with a lower quality of life and come with their own list of new symptoms to battle. However, often, it is still lifestyle measures that are the answer. Even though the overall descriptions of root causes of health are the same - the details can have a big impact. And these minor adjustments can make all the difference for the individual. We are, unique and our roads to healing are unique.

In this complex picture, some of us will benefit from finding and working with a health care practitioner to get on the right track.

You may also see the debut of new symptoms such as increased fatigue, weight loss, mental and cognitive abilities change or disruption of bowel habits. Then there is definitely time to get a check-up from your doctor.

How to find a health care practitioner

Chemistry is important when working with a health care practitioner. If you do not feel that you are listened to or taken seriously, you will not open up about symptoms or get the help you need. Here is what you can do to improve communication with your doctor:

Prepare before the visit. What do you want your doctor to learn about you and how you are feeling? What questions do you have for your doctor? Write it down if you need to and bring it to your visit.

Back up your claims with references. Doctors have no way of learning about all the new research being done. Bring relevant references for them to learn more about why want to try certain things in your treatment.

If that does not work, you know what? You may change doctors until you find someone who will listen and take your concerns seriously.

Finding a practitioner experienced in integrative medicine

Practitioners in conventional medicine may be fantastic at seeing the whole patient and not just looking at the lab result to see how you "should" feel. They listen and are open to suggesting alternatives to the first line of treatment for thyroid autoimmune disease. Other times, it may feel like speaking to a wall trying to be heard when you say that despite perfect levels of TSH, T4 or whatever, you still do not feel well. In that case, an integrative health care practitioner may be for you. Often, they are trained to use a holistic approach and think outside of the lab test/drug treatment box.

It is impossible to know where in the world you who are reading this are located. Each region and country has their own licenses and certifications for integrative practitioner. Traditional Chinese medicine, Ayurveda, and functional medicine are examples of integrative medical approaches common in different parts of the world.

If you are in the US, you may find an integrative practitioner via American Board of Integrative Medicine, American Board of Integrative and Holistic Medicine, or IFM - Institute of Functional Medicine. IFM also certify international practitioner and it can be worth looking in their practitioner directory even if you do not live in US. If you join Facebook Groups dedicated to Graves', women will happily share what doctors they successfully work with. Always confirm the level of training of your practitioner and ask for details on the treatments, tests or supplements they suggest.

NOTES

This is a selection of key references. You will find the complete, extensive medical and scientific bibliography for free at www.healinggravesbook.com.

Abbott RD, S. A. (2019). Efficacy of the Autoimmune Protocol Diet as Part of a Multi-disciplinary, Supported Lifestyle Intervention for Hashimoto's Thyroiditis. Cureus, 11(4):e4556.

Abraham-Nordling M, B. K. (2011). Incidence of Hyperthyroidism in Sweden. J Endocrinol, 2011;165(6):899–905.

Abraham-Nordling M, T. O. (2005). Graves' disease: a long-term quality-of-life follow up of patients randomized to treatment with antithyroid drugs, radioiodine, or surgery. . Thyroid, 15:1279- 86.

Boelaert K, N. P. (2010). Prevalence and relative risk of other autoimmune diseases in subjects with autoimmune thyroid disease. The American journal of medicine,123(2), 183.e1–183.e1839.

Bonaz B, B. T. (2018). The Vagus Nerve at the Interface of the Microbiota-Gut-Brain Axis. . Front Neurosci., 2018;12:49. . 3 Bordoni B, P. S. (2018). The Influence of Breathing on the Central Nervous System. Cureus, 2018;10(6):e2724.

Bouzas EA, K. P. (2000;). Antioxidant agents in the treatment of Graves' ophthalmopathy. Am J Ophthalmol. , 129(5):618–622.

Brüll F, M. R. (2010). TLR2 activation is essential to induce a Th1 shift in human peripheral blood mononuclear cells by plant stanols and plant sterols. J Biol Chem. , 2010;285(5):2951-2958.

Bustle. (2019).https://www.bustle.com/p/7-signs-you-have-low-grade-inflammation-whyyou-should-pay-attention-to-it-16102033

Cramer, H. L. (2012). Mindfulness-based stress reduction for breast cancer– a systematic review and meta-analysis. Current Oncology, , 19(5), e343-e352.

Cuciureanu MD, V. R. (2011). Magnesium and stress. In: Vink R, Nechifor M, editors. Magnesium in the Central Nervous System [Internet]. Adelaide (AU): University of Adelaide Press; 2011.

Cusick MF, L. J. (2012). Molecular mimicry as a mechanism of autoimmune disease. Clin Rev Allergy Immunol. , 42(1):102–111.

Cutovic M, K. L.-P. (2012). Structured exercise program improves functional capacity and delays relapse in euthyroid patients with Graves' disease. Disabil Rehabil., 2012;34(18):1511–1518.

D., K. (2017). The Role of Vitamin D in Thyroid Diseases. Int J Mol Sci, 18(9):1949. Published 2017 Sep 12.

Daimon CM, C. P. (2013). The role of Thyrotropin Releasing Hormone in aging and neurodegenerative diseases. . Am J Alzheimers Dis (Columbia)., (1):10.7726/ajad.2013.1003.

Danielsen ER, E. T. (2008). Reduced parietooccipital white matter glutamine measured by proton magnetic resonance spectroscopy in treated graves' disease patients.. J Clin Endocrinol Metab, 2008;93(8):3192–3198.

De Couck M, C. R. (2019;). How breathing can help you make better decisions: Two studies on the effects of breathing patterns on heart rate variability and decision-making in business cases. Int J Psychophysiol, 139:1-9.

de Menezes KJ, P. C. (2016;12:24–37.). Dehydroepiandrosterone, Its Sulfate and Cognitive Functions. . Clin Pract Epidemiol Ment Health. . Dekker JM, C. R. (2000). Low heart rate variability in a 2-minute rhythm strip predicts risk of coronary heart disease and mortality from several causes: the ARIC Study. Atherosclerosis Risk In Communities. Circulation., 2000;102(11):1239–1244.

Effraimidis, G. (2012). Early stages of thyroid autoimmunity: follow-up studies in the Amsterdam AITD cohort . PhD thesis.

Effraimidis, G. (2019). MANAGEMENT OF ENDOCRINE DISEASE: Predictive scores in autoimmune thyroid disease: are they useful? Eur J Endocrinol., 2019;181(3):R119–R131.

Elberling TV, D. E.-R. (2003). Reduced myo-inositol and total choline measured with cerebral MRS in acute thyrotoxic Graves' disease. Neurology, 2003;60(1):142–145.

Elias PK, E. M. (2005). Serum cholesterol and cognitive performance in the Framingham Heart Study. Psychosom Med., 67(1):24–30.

Espinosa-Diez C, M. V. (2015). Antioxidant responses and cellular adjustments to oxidative stress.. Redox Biol, 2015;6:183-197. F,

B. J. (2018). The hygiene hypothesis in autoimmunity: the role of pathogens and commensals. Nature reviews. Immunology,, 105–120.

Ferreira GC, M. M. (2017). L-Carnitine and Acetyl-L-carnitine Roles and Neuroprotection in Developing Brain. Neurochem Res., 2017;42(6):1661–1675.

Glintborg D, R. K. (2019). Increased risk of thyroid disease in Danish women with polycystic ovary syndrome: a cohort study. Endocr Connect. , 2019;8(10):1405–1415.

Golubić M, S. D. (2018). Comprehensive Lifestyle Modification Intervention to Improve Chronic Disease Risk Factors and Quality of Life in Cancer Survivors. Altern Complement Med, ;24(11):1085–1091.

Graham CD, G. J. (2016). A systematic review of the use of Acceptance and Commitment Therapy (ACT) in chronic disease and long-term conditions. . Clin Psychol Rev. , 2016;46:46–58.

Hölzel BK, C. J. (2011). Mindfulness practice leads to increases in regional brain gray matter density. Res., 191(1):36–43.

Inatsuki B, H. M. (1973). Studies on the biochemical properties of human thyroid gland mitochondria. . J Biochem. , 74(4):837-848.

Ji, D. P. (2018). Comparative assessment of Graves' disease and main extrathyroidal manifestation, Graves' ophthalmopathy, by non-targeted metabolite profiling of blood and orbital tissue. Sci Rep 8, 9262 .

Kahaly GJ, P. F. (2005). . Psychosocial Morbidity of Graves' Orbitopathy. Clin Endocrinol , 63(4):395- 402.

Lounassalo I, H. M. (2019). Associations of Leisure-Time Physical Activity Trajectories with Fruit and Vegetable Consumption from Childhood to Adulthood: The Cardiovascular Risk in Young Finns Study. . Int J Environ Res Public Health., 16(22):4437.

M, H. (2020). Outcome of Graves' disease. Thesis. M., G. (2014). Soy and legume seeds as sources of isoflavones: selected individual determinants of their consumption in a group of perimenopausal women. Prz Menopauzalny, 13(1):27–31.

M., N. (2015). Possible role of glial cells in the relationship between thyroid dysfunction and mental disorders. Front Cell Neurosci, 2015;9:194. Published 2015 Jun 3.

Osman F, F. J. (2007). Cardiovascular manifestations of hyperthyroidism before and after antithyroid therapy: a matched case-control study. . J Am Coll Cardiol., 2007;49(1):71–81.

P., K. (2003). Th1/Th2 balance: the hypothesis, its limitations, and implications for health and disease. . Altern Med Rev., 2003;8(3):223-246.

P., L. (2006). Remission of Graves' disease during anti-thyroid drug therapy. Time to reconsider the mechanism? Eur J Endocrinol., 155(6):783–786.

Ryödi E, M. S. (2018). Cardiovascular Morbidity and Mortality After Treatment of Hyperthyroidism with Either Radioactive Iodine or Thyroidectomy [published correction appears in . Thyroid. , 2018 Dec;28(12):1731

Salvatore D, S. W. (2014). Thyroid hormones and skeletal muscle--new insights and potential implications. Nat Rev Endocrinol, 10(4):206–214.

Sjölin G, H. M. (2019). The Long-Term Outcome of Treatment for Graves' Hyperthyroidism. Thyroid, 29(11):1545–1557.

Törpel A, H. F. (2018). Strengthening the Brain-Is Resistance Training with Blood Flow Restriction an Effective Strategy for Cognitive Improvement?. J Clin Med.

Törring O, W. T. (2019). Impaired Quality of Life After Radioiodine Therapy Compared to Antithyroid Drugs or Surgical Treatment for

Graves' Hyperthyroidism: A Long-Term Follow-Up with the Thyroid-Related Patient-Reported Outcome Questionnaire and 36-Item Short Form Health Status . Thyroid, ;29(3):322–331.

Urbańska B, K. J. (2019). Comparison of the Total Polyphenol Content and Antioxidant Activity of Chocolate Obtained from Roasted and Unroasted Cocoa Beans from Different Regions of the World. Antioxidants, 8(8):283.

Vaitkus JA, F. J. (2015). Thyroid Hormone Mediated Modulation of Energy Expenditure. Int J Mol Sci., 16(7):16158-16175.

Yuan L, T. Y. (2015). Decision-Making in Patients with Hyperthyroidism: A Neuropsychological Study. . PLoS One, 10(6):e0129773.

Yuksel N, Y. D. (2020;). The Effect of Smoking on Mitochondrial Biogenesis in Patients With Graves Ophthalmopathy. Ophthalmic Plast Reconstr Surg. , 36(2):172-177.

Zhao F, F. J. (2018). Alterations of the Gut Microbiota in Hashimoto's Thyroiditis Patients. Thyroid, ;28(2):175–186.

ACKNOWLEDGEMENTS

I want to thank the following people for help when this book becomes a reality:

Kerstin Brismar, Karl Hultén, Petra Kalla, Mia Lundin, Gunilla Saupe, Anna Sparre and Ove Törring who have generously contributed their time and knowledge.

All of you who have contributed your stories about your own health journeys. So many wise people I have had the honour of listening to and learning from.

Researchers and everyone all professionally working with health who dedicate their time and energy to gaining more knowledge about Graves'.

Joel, my husband, thank you for everything you have given me. I do not even want to think about what my life would have been like without you. And thanks for the expert advice on physical activity.

Teodor and Siri, my children. It was the desire to become a more energetic mother that drove me further on the quest to regain my quality of life. In the end it worked and now I can come along for all the fun again.

Stina, mother-in-law, because you are always positive about my projects and ideas. It is invaluable to be encouraged before a step into the unknown. And for the proofreading.

And thanks to you the reader, the reason for writing this book is to help you understand your condition better.

INDEX

Printed in Great Britain
by Amazon

46837144R00162